T5-AFU-034

Destroy the
Mask.
Carla O'Reily

Adjust your Sail
Tania
Bird

The Smiling Mask

Truths about Postpartum Depression and Parenthood

It's time to learn
from JOY...instead
of pain!
Elita Paterson
xo

Copyright © 2008 by To the Core Consulting
Carla O'Reilly, Elita Paterson and Tania Bird

All rights reserved. No part of this work may be reproduced or transmitted in any form or by any means – graphic, electronic or mechanic, including photocopying, recording, taping or information storage and retrieval systems – without the prior written permission of the publisher, or in the case of photocopying or other reprographic copying, a license from the Canadian Copyright Licensing Agency.

All health and health-related information contained in this book is intended to be general in nature and does not reflect all treatment options. No information in this book may be considered as medical advice. To the Core Consulting and Purpose to Prosperity Publishing assumes no responsibility for how you use information obtained in this book. Before making any decisions regarding your health care, ask a qualified health professional.

Library and Archives Canada Cataloguing in Publication

THE SMILING MASK – Truths about Postpartum Depression and Parenthood
By Carla O'Reilly, Elita Paterson, Tania Bird, and Peggy Collins
Includes bibliographical references.
ISBN 978-0-9781341-3-6

1. Postpartum depression – Popular works. 2. Postpartum depression – Patients – Biography. 3. Postpartum depression – Patients – Family relationships. I. O'Reilly, Carla, 1977

RG852.S65 2008   618.7'6   C2008-904796-6

Cover and Layout Design: Jay Roach
Editor: Peggy Collins
Contributing Editor: Marlene Harper PhD (Psych), MA (C. Psych)
Group Photo: Bishop Weber Photography

Published by:
Purpose to Prosperity Publishing
3033 Victoria Ave, Regina, Saskatchewan S4T 1L1 Canada

www.thesmilingmask.com

Printed and bound in Canada

Purpose to Prosperity Publishing
gratefully acknowledges the financial assistance of the
Saskatchewan Publishers Group through the
Cultural Industries Development Fund

The Smiling Mask

Truths about Postpartum Depression and Parenthood

* * *

Carla O'Reilly, Elita Paterson, Tania Bird and Peggy Collins

Praise for "The Smiling Mask"

"Courage, grace, hope and humour are gifts you are giving other women on similar journeys. Thank you for having the courage to share your story."

~ Justine

"What a creative and courageous contribution to women's health; and what a valuable resource for so many other women and their friends and families. For far too long, Postpartum Depression has been shrouded in silence and shame. These stories from women who have lived with this, offers hope, insights and a sense of 'good mothering' so that other mothers don't feel so alone and lonely."

~ Margaret McKinnon, PhD

"It was very courageous and vulnerable and I was proud to know you as I read it. I felt you handled everything, especially other people, in the story with integrity and sensitivity. My heart broke for you as I imagined the isolation you felt in your darkness, but your story is full of hope and light."

~ Jackie Ludke, mother of three children

"My rating... excellent! Sincerely heart felt, and uplifting in spite of the fact that the story is about you at your worst. I'll say that again ... Uplifting, that is the tone I felt throughout, and gently spiritual. Congratulations on the gift you are giving others."

~ Danita

"WOW!!! Bravo! Bravo! I couldn't stop reading. I cried and I laughed. You told it like it was and it is. But for the Grace of God, neither I nor any of my closest girlfriends has experienced POSTPARTUM DEPRESSION, but one never knows when they might need the valuable information you are offering... we all have daughters."

~ Colleen Oshowy, R.N.

"I love the fairytale that begins the book. In many ways it actually reminded me of myself. I think we all do that at times, put on the mask, knowing that eventually we have to take it off and really begin to look at ourselves. I have found that anger and fear and guilt make you ugly. You can either cover it up or let it control your life, or throw out that mask and let go of those feelings. Eventually that beautiful person shines through!"

~ Jamie Warwick – mother of twins

To the Core Consulting
&
Purpose to Prosperity Publishing

… are pleased to donate $1.00 from every sale of

"The Smiling Mask"

Shared equally to the following charitable organizations:

Women's Shelters – Carla chose this charity because she recognizes how some mothers and women are trapped in a world of violence and require assistance. Women's shelters support women and children in crisis.

YMCA/YWCA – Elita chose this charity because she recognizes the importance of postpartum support groups, which these organizations provide, as well as providing excellent childcare to assist mothers who return to the workforce.

NICU/Mother and Baby Ward – Tania chose this charity because she acknowledges the loving care that was given to Katherine, her daughter, who required a several month stay in the NICU. Tania had a six week stay within the Mother and Baby Ward. Both wards play key roles in saving lives.

Canadian Mental Health Association – Peggy chose this charity because she recognizes the tremendous need to find solutions and increase the support required to assist families suffering from all forms of mental illness, and especially those with Postpartum Depression.

The Rising

Lost and so low, abandoned, slipping, sliding
Urgent screams cut freedom out of the night,
Smother, smother thinks the mother
Oh, so dark has gone the night.

Chubby legs running, arms open, inviting
Golden sunlight on beaming, sweet eyes
I love you, Mommy, whispers the child
Oh, so quick the dream has died.

I hear you dear child from down in my dungeon
I hear you my love, I'll find the strength to rise,
How can I tell you how much I love you?
How can I tell you the dark thoughts I hide?

Chubby hands tugging with endless demanding
Milk on the floor feels like mud in my eye,
How do I handle this constant annoyance?
How do I live when I want to die?

Rise with me child
We'll run to the sunlight,
I'll love you forever
I'll clear the mist from my eyes.

You are my baby,
My one and my only,
Deep down in my heart
I know we'll survive.

Charmaine Korchynski, April 16, 2008
Dedicated to the courageous women who battle and recover from Postpartum Depression.

Contents

Foreward

Donna Bowyer

Branch Director
Canadian Mental Health Association
Moose Jaw Branch

I am honoured to be a part of this remarkable book, The Smiling Mask - Truths about Postpartum Depression and Parenthood, where three very brave women bring their experience, knowledge, strength and message of hope on a subject, which like other mental illnesses has remained a secret. This secret has resulted in women, their husbands and families struggling in silence.

Carla, Tania and Elita have the courage to share their very personal story of their struggle with Postpartum Depression (PPD) each with her own insights. There is no magic formula that will see you through, but having the courage to 'fight the fight' and know that there is hope is an inspiration to those with PPD, their partners and their families.

For every woman, having a baby is a challenging time, both mentally and physically. It is important for women to have the information to be able to know that if they are one of the women that is struggling with Postpartum Depression to first know that it is not their fault and that it does not reflect on their value as a mother, or a person, and that there is help and hope.

There is nobody exempt from the possibility of having this illness. No circumstances, wealth, education, preparedness, or status can insure that you will not struggle with Postpartum Depression. In an article in Anchor

Magazine, Amy Sky (singer, songwriter) tells about her struggle with both of her pregnancies. She says she was "...waiting for normal." That didn't work for her, as it didn't for Carla, Tania and Elita. They realized that they had to do something so other people would not have to struggle as they had.

Each woman that struggles has her own story. Each of the three women and their families has a unique story to tell of their journey toward recovery. There are, however, some things that are common for people with Postpartum Depression; detachment from life, exhaustion, confusion and fear. Many also struggle with despair so profound that they contemplate suicide.

I know that within these pages you will find enlightenment and admiration for these women and their husbands and the courage it has taken them to "fight the fight" and to bring their story to you in hopes that someday everyone will be prepared and have the tools to deal with this illness.

Just as your body can be traumatized by physical changes in childbirth so can your mind. Those that struggle are not alone, there is help, and Carla, Tania and Elita will share with you where they found help and hope.

Sally Elliott

R.N. Perinatal Nurse Counsellor
YMCA of Regina

There are myriad of biological, chemical, hormonal, psychological and social reasons for this illness. It can be caused by hormonal imbalances, sleep deprivation, isolation, traumatic pregnancy or birth, high needs babies, poverty or abuse – just to name a few.

It is particularly unfortunate that women feel ashamed and guilty when they have this illness. Many feel that they are "bad mothers" and that they have caused this disease because of things that they may have done wrong or failed to do. Some feel overwhelmed with feelings of hopelessness and worthlessness, while others can be consumed by anxiety and obsessive thoughts.

It helps everyone to talk honestly about Postpartum Depression and to bring them out into the open. Talking helps women to realize that they are not alone and that they will get better. Women need to hear and understand that they are good mothers who have a treatable illness.

Medical professionals, counsellors and social workers are all very helpful for these women, but I also feel that women sharing their stories, feelings, experiences and suggestions with each other, can be the most helpful resource of all! Sharing together normalizes feelings, allows expression of concerns, gives opportunity for discussion and suggests tools and resources for health.

For all these reasons, I believe that Elita, Tania and Carla's book is very welcomed, timely and most needed. I am grateful for their concern and empathy; I applaud their honesty and I am proud to know them. Women can take much comfort and wisdom from their words.

Preface
Postpartum Depression Explained

Marlene Harper, PhD

(Psych), MA (Clinical Psych)
Registered Psychologist, APE (@MA)

The world is full of suffering. It is also full of the overcoming it.
~ Helen Keller

The birth of a new baby is an event of joy, celebration, pride and love. The pregnant mother often day-dreamed about how she would love, nurture, protect and care for her precious baby. Life would be wonderful! Excited anticipation brought images of basking in love, rocking her baby to sleep, cuddling with her baby and partner while feeling a renewed closeness and intimacy and showing her or him off with pride to all her family and friends. Unfortunately, many mothers feel like crying and dying instead of celebrating. The authors of "The Smiling Mask" have bravely shared their stories, their truths, and the feelings they experienced when they suffered Postpartum Depression (PPD) after the birth of their first child. Removing their "masks" and telling others about their illness facilitated their healing. Sharing their story has been personally cathartic and validating for them but has had a wider impact than they would have expected. During and after their public presentations; (a) women have cried in relief and support, (b) families have been inspired to be more empathic, and (c) professionals have reported their resolve to listen and question mothers about their symptoms, use screening evaluations, and improve prevention and intervention strategies for PPD.

PPD is much more than "baby blues" or feeling fatigued and overwhelmed with the myriad of responsibilities and adjustments (physiological, social and behavioural) after having a baby. Most women cope, adjust and thrive. However, when a person is clinically depressed, the symptoms last at least two weeks, and are so extensive and distressing that they interfere with social, occupational and other important areas of functioning. Symptoms may vary and the severity of the symptoms is not the same in each person and can range from mild, moderate to severe. It is a state of persistent depressed mood and loss of interest or pleasure that occurs together with other physical and mental symptoms, such as insomnia or excessive sleep, appetite disturbance, excessive unproductive body activity (e. g., pacing, tapping, etc.) or slowing down of body activity, movement and speech and fatigue, weight loss or gain, poor concentration and feelings of guilt, worthlessness, hopelessness, helplessness, and thoughts of death [1]. PPD can interfere with a mother's ability to take care of herself and her newborn baby. Some women can "go through the motions," but in the most severe situations suicide can occur, psychosis can develop, and in rare circumstances it can result in infanticide.

PPD is not new and women have gone through this for centuries but the negative consequences for the mother, infant and family should not be dismissed [2]. PPD reduces the mother's social adjustment, self-esteem and quality of life and marital conflict is also common when mothers are depressed [3,4,5]. Researchers have suggested that infants and children whose mothers are depressed, especially if PPD is chronic, are at risk for (a) impaired cognitive and language development, (b) emotional problems (e. g., lower self-esteem, anxiety, fearfulness, sadness, passivity and dependency), (c) social problems (e. g., insecure relationships, detachment, social withdrawal or aggression), and (d) behaviour problems (e. g., sleep disruption, temper tantrums, fussiness, tearfulness, aggression and hyperactivity) [6,7,8,9,10,11,12,13,14,15,16,17,18,19,20,21]. Persistent or chronic PPD could lead to insecure mother-infant attachment or bonding [13] and negative mother-infant interactions [11,12]. Long lasting and recurring PPD is also associated with adolescent externalizing disorders such as conduct disorder and aggression [22,23,24,25], and psychiatric and medical disorders [7,15,16,22,23,24,25].

It is also common for fathers to become depressed when mothers are depressed [26] which can further increase the mother's depression and in turn, the baby's development [27,28]. Yet, fathers' depression can also be independent of PPD. Depressed fathers have a negative impact on children's emotional development and behaviour including an increased risk of conduct problems in boys [28]. Fathers who have depression or anxiety may be at increased risk to use abuse alcohol and drugs [18,28,30] which adds further personal and family stresses [27]. It doesn't mean that mothers are the cause of fathers' depression; it means that men may also be unable to cope with the adjustments, changing roles, demands and expectations of parenthood and the added stresses that occur when their partner has PPD.

Although there are negative and disastrous effects of PPD for women and their families, the good news is that depression is one of the most researched and successfully treated mental health disorders [31]. Treatment that is specific to improving parenting practices and mother-child interactions can improve cognitive development [16]. In some people, clinical depression goes away on its own without medical intervention, many months later [1], perhaps because the person solved some of their problems, improved coping skills and used their social supports. Women don't choose to have PPD. The symptoms are outside their control and they should not be blamed, but by getting help they can control how they cope. Women with PPD suffer tremendous guilt and shame. They commonly try to hide the symptoms because they fear (a) the stigma associated with mental health, (b) being judged, and (c) losing their babies. Women may also simply think the symptoms are temporary because they are adjusting to physical, social and behavioural changes in their lives [32]. Depression does not result from a character flaw and it is not a sign of weakness. Acknowledging that she is not coping and asking for help takes courage and strength; it is one of the least selfish things a woman with PPD may ever do.

Only qualified mental health professionals (i. e., physicians, psychiatrists, and clinical psychologists) may diagnose PPD after completing a clinical diagnostic interview with the mother. PPD is not considered a separate illness but is part of an affective or mood disorder [1]. It is usually a Major Depressive Disorder (MDD), commonly called "clinical depression," which occurs postpartum. Diagnosis is complicated and a person should not diagnose themselves. It may be difficult to distinguish between what may be seemingly "normal" reactions to childbirth and symptoms of depression [33]. Some medical conditions (e. g., anemia, thyroid dysfunction, etc.) are similar to those in clinical depression and can occur together with depression or must be ruled out. Drug reactions or drug and alcohol abuse must also be ruled out. The symptoms may be a due to a different psychiatric disorder and more than one diagnosis may also be given (e. g., an anxiety disorder, substance abuse, etc.). In some situations, bereavement may better account for the symptoms [1].

Different mental illnesses, including Major Depressive Disorder, Bipolar Disorder or Brief Psychotic Episode, can be diagnosed and specified as having a postpartum onset if the symptoms present within the first four weeks postpartum and last at least two weeks [1]. However, the symptoms of PPD can be the most severe many months later. Some researchers [33] suggest that PPD could be diagnosed if the woman has a depressive episode that occurs within the first year postpartum. Others state that PPD should be considered if depressive symptoms occur within 6 months after birth [21]. Symptoms usually start within the first 12 weeks postpartum [33]. Other psychiatric disorders may also develop and be diagnosed after birth (e. g., Post-Traumatic Stress Disorder, other anxiety disorders, etc.) [1,33,35]. As well, symptoms of previous psychiatric disorders can increase [33,35].

The number of people affected by Major Depressive Disorder (MDD) is staggering [43]. About 10% to 25% of women and 5% to 12% of men will suffer MDD at some time in their lives. At any one time, 5% to 9% of women and 2% to 3% of men are suffering MDD [1]. The highest rates of clinical depression occur in women during the reproductive years [2] and depression is the most frequent disorder after childbirth [35]. Therefore, "the postpartum period is considered a time of increased risk for the onset of mood disorders." [33, p. 15] PPD affects approximately 13% of new mothers [38]. Unfortunately, if a woman has had PPD, there is a 50% chance of reoccurrence [38,40].

Women with PPD may have similar symptoms but they can vary in occurrence and severity. Some women have weak social supports and inadequate coping skills. Childhood traumas, family-of-origin conflicts and negative parenting can reduce coping and leave people vulnerable when dealing with adult stressors. Negative reactions to drugs, drug or alcohol abuse, physical illness and stress (e. g., complicated bereavement, loss of job, childbirth, relationship breakup, work stress, lower socioeconomic disadvantage and the time for year for some people) can precipitate clinical depression [7, 33]. Whenever one tragic or multiple stressful events or losses mount up and are more than our resources or ability to cope, we can get depressed. Whenever our safety, security, integrity and identity are threatened and we are unable to cope, we can get depressed.

A complex interaction, a biopsychosocial model, is often used to explain depression and other mental illnesses. In the biopsychosocial model, multiple domains, not just one, contribute to mental health problems for example; (a) biological factors can include genetic predispositions, medical problems or illness, and/or biochemical imbalances, (b) psychological or mental factors entails thoughts, emotions and behaviours, and (c) social aspects involve the social, relationship and the cultural environment (e. g., social support, relationship loss, women's role in society, etc.) [34]. Therefore, treatment using a biopsychosocial perspective may involve medication management and exercise, changing irrational negative thought patterns, and encouraging improving the mother's social supports.

There is much controversy in the scientific literature about what precipitates PPD [35], and as stated earlier, the cause of PPD remains unclear [33]. A hormonal basis has been considered but research has not found a specific hormone associated with PPD [33]. Women who are most vulnerable to PPD are those with (a) previous psychiatric disorders, especially depression and anxiety themselves or in their family [36,37], (b) poor social supports [31], (c) marital problems, (d) life stress, (e) a higher amount of stress during pregnancy [27,31,33,35], and (f) social disadvantage [38,39]. Stress during pregnancy can include a difficult delivery, prenatal problems, premature birth, or illness during pregnancy [33]. Anxiety and negative experiences during pregnancy and anxiety about birth can be predictive of psychiatric and depressive symptoms postpartum [35]. Although not conclusive, there may be a hormonal sensitivity and biochemical involvement in PPD [2,38] such as a history of severe PMS or premenstrual dysphoric disorder [33]. Rapid hormonal changes (e. g., estrogen, progesterone, etc.) may also trigger PPD [33].

Psychiatric symptoms after childbirth are usually clustered into (a) Postpartum Blues, (b) Postpartum Depression, and (c) Postpartum Psychosis [35].

Postpartum Blues
The research indicates that 15% to 85% of women may experience "baby blues" which often begins immediately postpartum and remits within days [41,33]. The wide variance in percentage may be due to different methodologies used in the studies. "Baby blues" are most likely caused by hormonal changes following birth [21]. The symptoms usually peak at 5 days and remit by 7 to 10 days [41]. Symptoms may include a lack of emotional stability, mood swings, irritability, fatigue, tearfulness, generalized anxiety, sleep and appetite disturbance, confusion, mild manic symptoms and elation [18,33,41]. Postpartum blues are temporary, mild, time-limited and do not require treatment other than support and reassurance because they reduce on their own without medical intervention [42]. However, they can be a risk factor for PPD [2,42]. Approximately 20% of women with postpartum blues develop PPD but other women may do well after childbirth and then PPD may gradually develop later [33].

Postpartum Depression
Non-psychotic PPD begins in the postpartum period. Symptoms can come on suddenly right after childbirth or several months to a year later [38,33]. The

DSM-IV criteria, which mental health professionals use to make a diagnosis, are the most stringent at 4 weeks postpartum. Although individual studies indicate that PPD ranges from 6% to 22%, these differences are due to different methodologies and diagnostic criteria used [35]. It is more accepted that approximately 13% of new mothers experience PPD [38]. The symptoms are similar to clinical depression unrelated to childbirth and not classified as a separate mental illness [1]. As well, mothers with PPD often worry excessively about the baby's health, well-being and safety and may have intrusive thoughts about harming the baby, but acting on the thought is rare. Lack of concentration, psychomotor agitation (e. g., pacing, wringing hands, pulling clothing off and on, excessively chewing fingernails, etc.) or retardation (e. g., slowing down of body movement, speech, etc.) and suicide thoughts are common. Severe anxiety, panic attacks, spontaneous crying, insomnia and disinterest in the baby are also prominent in PPD. Many women with PPD feel overwhelming guilt at a time when they believe that they should be happy [1]. Low self-esteem, inability to cope, loneliness, feeling incompetent and loss of self also contributes and exacerbates PPD [33].

Postpartum Psychosis

PPD may include psychotic features, a loss of contact with reality, which usually includes (a) delusions (i. e., unshakeable false paranoid or irrational ideas or beliefs about what is taking place or who one is) and (b) hallucinations (i. e., seeing things that are not there or hearing voices). Delusions are an abnormality in a person's thoughts, and hallucinations involve the senses. Psychosis can occur in medical, neurological and mental health disorders. It is a medical emergency and hospitalization is usually necessary to stabilize the symptoms and keep both the mother and baby safe [21]. PPD psychosis is uncommon but severe and there is a high risk for suicide and infanticide [21]. It effects approximately 1 in 500 to 1 in 1000 deliveries and most common in the first delivery [1,33].

Postpartum psychosis occurs rapidly with symptoms sometimes escalating within 48 hours and it can be difficult to predict. Episodes can present as early as 48 to 72 hours postpartum but most often begin within the first two weeks, yet can also present later [33]. Women with Postpartum psychosis can appear well, thus health professionals and the family may believe she has recovered, only to soon find that she suddenly becomes severely depressed or psychotic [45]. As well, she may be paranoid and not show or tell others about her symptoms, therefore making it difficult for health professions to evaluate or predict the escalation of the illness. Early warning signs include an inability to sleep, agitation, euphoria or irritability, and avoidance of the baby [21]. Depressed or elated mood, which can fluctuate rapidly, disorganized behaviour, extreme anxiety, agitation, confusion, bizarre behaviour, inability or refusal to eat or sleep, suicidal thoughts or actions, labile or unstable mood, thoughts of harming or killing the baby, delusions and hallucinations are common [1]. Postpartum psychosis resembles a manic episode and Bipolar Disorder can be a risk factor for development of PPD with psychosis [33].

When delusions are present in PPD, they usually are about the baby (e. g., believing the baby may be possessed, have special powers or be destined for a terrible fate) [1]. Not all mothers who have thoughts of harming or killing their baby will do so. It may be that the mother is afraid that she will contaminate the baby in some way by her presence and avoids contact. Infanticide is rare and although it can occur without hallucinations, it is usually associated with PPD psychosis when there may be command hallucinations to kill the baby or delusions that the baby is possessed. Unfortunately, PPD with psychotic episodes tends to reoccur in 30% to 50% of second births [1].

Treatment

Although there is a high incidence of clinical depression and PPD (approximately 13%), the intent of this brief summary is not to create anxiety or panic. Rather, it is to provide educational information so that women will be encouraged to seek help if they are unable to cope on their own. We must keep things in perspective. Some studies on depression have shown that although rates of depression may be as high as 17%, major depression accounted for 6.9%, minor depression, 1.8% and in the other 8.3%, depressive symptoms did not interfere with work or social functioning [43]. So, in that average of 13% of new mothers who develop PPD, there is a range of different severities of symptoms from mild, moderate to severe. Women have different genetics, symptoms, coping skills, and social supports which can either help buffer stress and increase coping or escalate stress and decrease coping. Children and families will be less impacted if the mother's symptoms are within the mild range of PPD. The earlier the intervention the better, but it is never too late to make changes. When people are in the depths of despair and when their life seems futile and hopeless, it is difficult to believe that life will get better but there is good potential for coping and healing. Women can begin healing by courageously removing their "mask" and asking for help.

Healthcare providers have a major role in screening and providing educational information, preventative practices, and interventions to reduce the occurrence of PPD and facilitate prevention and healing. Medical and psychological research is ongoing and necessary. Screening and identification of women with psychiatric disorders needs improvement as does removing barriers to accessible, acceptable and effective treatment [2]. Best Practice Guidelines have been developed [33] which can help with screening and intervention. There is a wealth of information in books, in the scientific literature and on credible internet sites for both professionals and consumers (e. g., The Registered Nurses' Association of Ontario www.rnao.org, www.helpguide.org, etc.). The authors of "The Smiling Mask" have described self-care interventions that they personally found useful. Most importantly, women must take the initiative for their own healthcare and healing. If depression is severe, then families may need to get her to her physician. Public health nurses and family physicians may be the mother's first contact, but women can also benefit from psychotherapy, support groups, applying self-help strategies and using their social supports.

PPD may be treated by antidepressants or other medications especially if PPD is severe or in combination with psychotherapy [44] or by psychotherapy alone. As stated earlier, Postpartum psychosis is a medical emergency and requires immediate medical intervention. "Antidepressant medication is the mainstay of treatment for moderate to severe PPD [45, p. 763]." Women who want to nurse their babies face a serious dilemma. Adverse effects in infants who are nursed when the mother uses antidepressants are rare. There is a suggestion that in some antidepressants, the levels of medication that reach the baby are low or undetectable. However, long term effects and the effect of trace amounts of medication are not known [2,33]. Unfortunately, untreated PPD can also result in devastating effects for her baby [2]. Women should consult with their physicians to help them make the best decision for themselves and their baby's medical and psychological health.

Psychotherapy is also effective in treating PPD. Cognitive Behavioural Therapy (CBT) and Interpersonal Therapy (IPT) are the most common and successful psychotherapies for the management of PPD even though more research is needed on the effectiveness of specific coping interventions [44]. CBT focuses on the importance of thoughts, beliefs, memories and emotions on behaviours. Clients are taught new adaptive and empowering ways to think and behave [46]. CBT psychotherapy is more than providing educational information, learning positive thinking and relaxation. It is a complex process whereby the psychotherapist facilitates changes in a woman's world view, beliefs, attitudes and behaviours in an empathic and supportive manner. It enhances cognitive skills, evaluation and modification of dysfunctional thoughts, and encourages self-regulation of emotions and behaviours, social skill development and using positive statements [2,46]. Interpersonal Therapy (IPT) focuses on relationships including marital relationships, role change, social support, and life stress. It is also often successful in the treatment of PPD [2,47].

Marriage counselling may also encourage the couple to work as a team and help navigate the many adjustments of parenting, improve communication and reduce marital conflict. Support groups that provide educational information, social support, validation and structure can also be helpful especially when severe depression is more stabilized. Learning educational information about parenting either from attending formal classes or by reading self-help books can reduce anxiety and frustration and can improve mother-infant interactions.

Lastly and most importantly, self-care and accepting help is essential after childbirth and in particular when coping with PPD. It is believed that some cultures have less PPD because they have strong social supports for new mothers such as help with childcare, providing of special foods, ritual baths, and even a short return to her family-of-origin [45]. We cannot control many events that occur, such as loss of a job or death of loved one, but we can learn to control how we react and cope. Managing stress begins by learning to control what we can and letting go of what we can't. People start by taking small steps not huge leaps. New mothers can help buffer stress by (a) reducing the number of stressful events or changes that they can (e. g., delaying remodeling the house until the next year), (b) using her social supports (e. g., avoiding isolation, joining a support group, asking family for help, setting up a mother's group in the neighborhood, meeting with her physician, or calling a therapist), (c) reducing extra responsibilities (e. g., the dust will wait, changing expectations, get help, etc.), (d) using positive thinking and affirmations even if you don't believe them yet (e. g., "This too will pass."), (e) eating healthy foods, exercising and resting, (f) taking time for herself, (g) using positive coping strategies such as talking to a friend rather than drinking, using drugs, or binging on alcohol or food, and (h) taking time for relaxation, meditation, prayer or just simply sighing to release body stress.

Removing "masks" is scary and can be terrifying because we then admit that we cannot do it alone and face the possibility of judgment. Yet, it is liberating and courageous. By removing her "mask," a new mother can find courage in adversity, strength in vulnerability, resiliency in trauma and hope in pain.

Introduction

"The Smiling Mask" is an inspirational book created to increase awareness, acceptance and assistance for those suffering with Postpartum Depression (PPD). The goal of the book is to shed light on the realities that many mothers and families face when their lives are affected by postpartum disorders. The women who struggle with PPD are often misunderstood and harshly judged. There is a critical need to raise awareness and provide support so that these families may flourish with joy and happiness, and ultimately reduce its negative effects on future generations. This book will enlighten mothers by giving hope and inner peace.

The book encompasses the lives of three women who have lived through the trauma of postpartum illnesses and who are willing to share their experiences and knowledge so that others may be helped. There is information that describes the agony the fathers/husbands/families endured. As well, there is self-help information to enlighten new mothers of potential warning signs. Symptoms and strategies are discussed to assist those who are currently experiencing postpartum illnesses and the people who support these mothers. Our vision and mission are as follows:

VISION

To inspire healing, hope and harmony for families.

MISSION

The purpose of "The Smiling Mask" is to create awareness, understanding, and acceptance of Postpartum Depression difficulties and to bring peace and validation to mothers by engaging and empowering families and communities in the life changing and natural experience of parenthood.

We believe passionately that a positive difference can be made. The outcome of sharing our stories will generate belief in motherhood by accepting PPD conditions and working together in community to make a positive difference for generations to come. Being afraid to speak up for assistance and remaining "silent" is a major characteristic that fuels the persistence of Postpartum Depression. As mothers we need to take responsibility for our health and seek help when we need it. This way we can transform our situations so that a healthier and happier world is created together. We believe that this healing starts with the mother.

We have found that writing our stories has enhanced our healing. We want to encourage those who are suffering with PPD to openly discuss their situation because they can then move forward and also heal. Our hope is that increased awareness and open communication will help women rise above their illness.

With heartfelt gratitude!

The Smiling Mask Team

Prologue – A Fairytale of the Perfect Mother

I awoke to the sound of my baby cooing in his crib. I arose from my bed and put on my mask. I slipped on my house coat, stepped into my baby's room and turned on the light. I picked up my baby and whispered soft words into his ears. I lovingly snuggled him. My little bundle needed his diaper changed, and so it was done. Now, everything was fresh and new. I was a perfect mother. I was cheerful and I remembered my appointment at 4:00 o'clock this afternoon.

I stepped into the kitchen and warmed a bottle for my little one. I smiled a beautiful smile and was ready for the day. I made coffee and sat down to watch my favourite morning talk show as I fed my little angel. I whispered sweet lullabies and spoke about all the things we would do together that day. I finished feeding him and grabbed a quick shower. My little boy played in the bouncy chair while listening to music. I remembered about my 4:00 o'clock appointment as I washed my hair.

I got dressed, blow dried my hair and put on my makeup. I then emptied the dishwasher and worked out a plan for supper. I chopped some vegetables and beef and put them in the slow cooker. My husband would be happy because it was his favourite meal. I planned to pick up some buns when I was out running errands. I was a perfect wife.

It was time to give my baby a bath. I gently washed his face and brushed his hair. Then I pulled out a new outfit which I purchased the day before. We got ready to go. I quickly packed the diaper bag and we headed out the door for a walk. Down the street we happily strolled. We waved and stopped to talk with the neighbour. The sun was shining, flowers were blooming and the birds were chirping. It was a beautiful day.

We walked downtown and stopped at the local grocery store for a few items; some eggs, buns, milk and butter. My baby drifted off to sleep by the time we met up with my friend and we continued to walk. We had a great visit. I had great friends and a perfect life.

I stopped in to see my husband at work and everyone tickled and played with the baby. Then our whole family went for lunch at the local café. The food tasted so good. I dropped off my baby with his grandmother while I went to have my hair styled at the local salon. I must look good for my 4:00 o'clock appointment. My hairdresser greeted me with fresh coffee and we gossiped for the next two hours. I got my hair coloured and set. It looked beautiful. I quickly said goodbye and headed home. I did not want to miss my appointment.

As I walked through the door of my house, I noticed the silence. I walked to the bathroom, went in and locked the door. I turned and looked into the mirror. I stared, and looked deeply at my face. There was always a smile, there was always a mask. I was terrified, yet determined. My appointment had come. It was time to deal with my relentless shame the best way I knew how. I felt like a monster and could take no more. It was time to end my life.

I knelt down on the floor, laid down in a fetal position and began to cry. Tears were streaming down my face. I didn't want to live with this painful secret. I loved my child so deeply and I began to feel his pain. I flashed to my funeral, watching my son so young, whispering goodbye to his mommy. I flashed to his first day of kindergarten, his high school graduation and his wedding. I flashed to my own mother who was breaking down sobbing and wondering what she could have done to help her daughter. I saw her walking the rest of her days with a shadow over her heart. I felt my family's pain resonate inside of me.

Then from somewhere, somehow a glimmer of hope rose up within me. I whispered to myself that the agony was going to end, but not through suicide. How close I was to dying; how necessary it seemed. I instead chose to remove the mask. Suddenly the pain, guilt and shame evaporated. I now had the courage to speak. There would be no more secrets! There would be no more lies! There would be no more smiling mask!

Greetings from

Elita, Carla and Tania

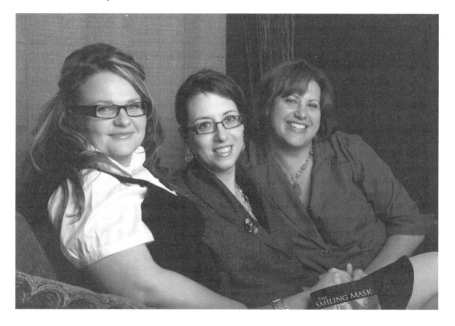

Here are our truths ....

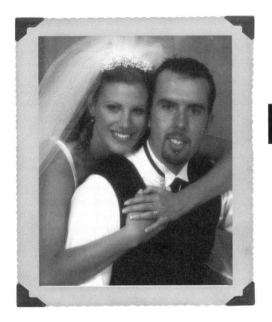

Carla's wedding photo

Carla after giving birth

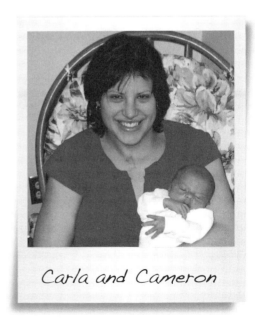

Carla and Cameron

Chapter One
Carla's Truth

If the eyes had no tears, the soul would have no rainbows.
~ First Nations proverb

You won't read about me in the headlines. You won't hear my tragic story on the evening news. My story is written for those who do not have a voice; women who are alone and too ashamed to speak. My struggle has not been without the help of many friends and strangers, who accepted me even when they knew the truth about my illness. They allowed me to realize that I wasn't an evil monster. I was just a mother who was unlucky.

It was late August 2004. I was in the Mental Health Ward of the Calgary Foothills Hospital, sitting with the doctor in a small, quiet room devoid of pictures or colour. The chair felt slightly uncomfortable and I was having trouble relaxing. There was a two-way mirror across from me and behind the mirror were unseen faces, writing and judging as I spoke. The doctor was a kind man who made me feel comfortable as he questioned me. "Tell us Carla, what brought you here?" As I spoke to the unseen faces, I began to remember what had happened to me eight months ago when my son, Cameron, was born.

I remembered the excitement we felt waiting as we tried the home pregnancy test. My husband, Curtis, and I were both in the bathroom as I urinated on the pregnancy strip, and waited the required five minutes for the results. We were so excited when it turned positive. We quickly phoned and shared the news with both sets of parents. I loved every moment of being pregnant because I was carrying our special baby! I started to imagine how I would decorate the nursery. I went shopping for maternity clothes. I wanted to look cute when my belly swelled.

In time, I could feel our little bundle moving around inside of me. I was so excited to feel the kicks and have Curtis feel them too. I loved being pregnant even though I was exhausted and towards the end, quite uncomfortable. When I was six months pregnant, I had a couple of scares where the doctor put me on bed rest because of early Braxton-Hicks contractions. We went for an ultrasound. When the doctor asked if we wanted to know the sex of the baby, Curtis excitedly said he would. I eagerly agreed and we found out it was a boy! When we were picking names we narrowed it down to two. Curtis liked Joseph and I favored Cameron. We decided Cameron Joseph would be fitting because both our initials were C. J.

We were able to sell our smaller house and purchase a larger home when I was six months pregnant in order to make room for our new addition. I was so excited to own a larger home. It didn't take me long to have the whole house packed. The weekend we were planning to move I was rushed to the hospital because of pain. The doctor confirmed that I was having early labour contractions and admitted me overnight. He decided I needed to be on bed rest for a week. Being on bed rest was boring, but at least I was being treated like a princess. People were attending to my every need.

Our friends helped us to move into the new house, which was a Godsend, because I was not able to do much strenuous work myself. The disarray and disorder in the house annoyed me. Curtis felt the same way and we actually did not know where to begin. My friend Kathy came over and in a matter of a few hours she had everything organized. This made me very happy. She even scrubbed our kitchen floor. My in-laws drove later that week to help us out as well from Moose Jaw, a small Saskatchewan city where Curtis and I grew up.

They unpacked boxes and hung pictures for us. Having people support you like this was so appreciated. Being parents-to-be is worrisome enough on its own but the added move only heightened my anxiety.

Living for four years in Oyen, a small town in Alberta of approximately 1000 people, taught us about community. There were always many hands willing to pitch in when someone needed help. We had many close friends and everyone supported each other. They demonstrated the true meaning of "it takes a village to raise a child." I will never forget our friends and the support they gave us. We often moved to different locations because of Curtis's work. Leaving those friends behind and starting fresh was difficult. When we visit their friendly faces are always welcoming and it is as if time stands still.

Our family home was becoming more complete each day. After the unpacking was done, one of our first tasks was to get Cameron's bedroom ready. We painted it a traditional blue and chose a Noah's Ark theme. I had already fallen in love with Cameron and would read to him and sing him lullabies while he cuddled in the womb. I read a few books on pregnancy, delivery and how to care for babies. I thought I was well prepared. Very few books mentioned Postpartum Depression (PPD). When I came across the little bits of information about PPD, I would generally skim over them, assuming it didn't apply to me. I thought that I could be sleep deprived or I may even experience the baby blues. Most certainly, I would not qualify for Postpartum Depression. I mistakenly thought I knew what to expect. There were no warnings. There was no mention of the struggles women had with this terrible depression. The mothers I knew never shared that they felt unhappy. As far as I knew, motherhood was a beautiful, exhilarating experience.

Curtis and I attended a prenatal class to learn about labour, delivery and breastfeeding. The public health nurses briefly discussed depression. Only limited information was given about services or medications that helped those experiencing severe symptoms. I believe there should have been more emphasis given about the statistics and types of symptoms women could experience.

According to the book "Conquering Postpartum Depression," 10 to 17 percent of women experience Postpartum Depression and the following contributes to PPD:

1) Depression or anxiety during pregnancy
2) Single parenting
3) Unplanned pregnancy
4) Unhappy marriage or relationship
5) Lack of social or emotional support
6) High-risk pregnancy
7) Traumatic life experiences during or after pregnancy
8) Traumatic labour and childbirth
9) Poverty, isolation, low education
10) A family history of mental illness including depression
11) Childhood abuse
12) Pre-natal mental health disorders

After the birth of a baby, women could experience Postpartum Depression, Post-traumatic Stress Disorder, Postpartum Obsessive-compulsive Disorder and the most severe, Postpartum Psychosis. [1] As I reflect on my life and my experiences with motherhood, there are clear events that put my struggles with this illness into motion. I could have never imagined that I would suffer from the worst possible condition, postpartum psychosis. I was a textbook case. How could this have happened? There are many possible answers. I will share the details with you, now.

My best friend Kathy was thirty-three weeks pregnant and eagerly awaiting the arrival of her new baby. We planned to do so much together as our babies grew. Kathy was about four months ahead of me in pregnancy and was able to give me some guidance. She offered advice about morning sickness, doctor appointments, maternity clothes, baby's growth and what kicks felt like. When I stopped by for a visit and a coffee, we sat next to each other and she told me that the baby was kicking and that I should touch her belly. I leaned over, put my hand on her stomach and felt it move. I couldn't wait to feel the strong kicks of my own child.

Kathy and I were starting on an exciting journey together. We looked forward to our children growing up together and being friends. My husband jokingly said that I lived in "La La Land" with sunshine and lollipops. He thought that my head was often somewhere in the clouds. I wanted to live out the fairytale of being a perfect mother who could handle anything and be content just like many of my friends who were already mothers. Nothing could have prepared me for the heartache that was about to develop, the sadness or the guilt. The memory of the past five years is as fresh in my mind as if they happened yesterday.

It was Thursday evening and I was working as a librarian at the local high school. Kathy called to chat and she sounded a little worried. She said that she hadn't felt much movement from her baby. I told her not to worry but to sit down and drink some juice just like it said in the book, "What to Expect When You're Expecting."[2] The juice would make the baby become active again or maybe it was just asleep. I tried to assure her that everything was fine. We made plans to meet for coffee that Friday afternoon.

I worked in the morning the next day, and then waited for Kathy to call after lunch. It was odd that she didn't call. I thought that maybe she and her husband decided to go shopping for a minivan in Medicine Hat, the closest major city to Oyen. I began to worry when I didn't hear from her that evening. I was tempted to call her mother but decided against it, because I didn't want to seem nosy. I went to bed feeling that something was wrong but dismissed it as over-worrying.

I noticed the display on the phone read Medicine Hat Hospital when I woke up the next morning. I quickly checked the phone and saw that someone had called several times. We shut the ringer off the previous night so that we could sleep in. I frantically asked Curtis to dial the number. Curtis talked to Trent, Kathy's husband, and he said that things weren't good. When Curtis told me to sit down, I knew that it was going to be bad news.

Kathy and I talked and she told me that her baby was dead. I was shocked and screamed, "No. This isn't fair and I'm so sorry!" We cried together over the phone. She explained that she would have to deliver the baby later that day. I couldn't understand why they could not just put her under anesthetic and do a caesarian section. The doctors wouldn't, saying that there was too much risk of infection. I wanted to drive to the hospital to be with her but she said it was best if I didn't. Her family was supporting her. I told her to be strong and that I would pray for her, Trent and the baby.

I was completely devastated and cried throughout the day and for the next few days. Kathy called me after the baby was stillborn to tell me it was a boy and they named him Jarett Samuel. Kathy and Trent spent some time with Jarett after the delivery. She said that they would be home on Monday and would give me a call then. I stayed home from work on Monday because I felt deeply sad and depressed. I was shocked and I couldn't shake the sick feeling I had in the pit of my stomach. Kathy called when she arrived home. I tried to sound positive but I had to hide the tears in my voice. I asked if I could visit her and she agreed.

I didn't know what to expect but there were several family members there when I arrived at Kathy's house. Trent, who is naturally quiet, was talking to his brother outside. I walked towards him not knowing what to say. We hugged and I whispered that I was sorry. Kathy greeted me at the door. She was sad but gave me a hug and a smile. We both cried and she said she wanted to show me the baby's footprint. We sat for awhile in the living room and cried some more. I felt guilty and awkward because I still had a baby and she didn't. I was experiencing what I now know is called survivor's guilt. They planned a small funeral for the immediate family. Kathy asked if Curtis and I would attend. I said, "Of course."

The next few days were a blur, yet I was able to stop by every day to drop off her mail and give her a hug. Everyone in town was quite saddened because Kathy is well liked. I feared that Kathy would have a hard time being around me but she told me that only other pregnant ladies bothered her. The day of the funeral came. Kathy's family came down the aisle at the church in succession with Kathy and Trent coming in last. Everyone tried to look strong but as we walked towards the small casket, the tears began to fall from everyone's eyes. No one wanted to say goodbye to this little angel. We received a small angel pin. Kathy's sister read from the Bible. "Lord, you have seen what is in my heart. You know all about me. Lord, even before I speak a word, you know all about it. You planned how many days I would live ... before I had lived through even one of them." Psalm 139: 1, 4, 16.

Kathy and Trent privately said goodbye to their baby while the rest of us walked to our vehicles. We all returned to Kathy's parent's house for coffee and a visit. I hugged Kathy and sat next to her. She looked strong, but a piece of her heart had been taken that day. I knew Kathy would need me more than ever and I vowed to be there for her. I took on her sadness and grieved with her. I helped her and listened whenever she needed to talk. I put myself in her shoes. I tried to imagine how she felt and to understand her pain.

A mother carrying a baby develops a special bond. Even before she knows the baby she begins to have hopes and dreams for the child and her family. When the baby dies there is hopelessness. A part of her is always missing. She always wonders what might have been. My friend is a very strong and giving person. After such loss and grief, she did not give up hope of having children and later had two healthy boys. Family is very important to her and her children are the most important thing in her life. She gives effortlessly and is a great mother. Mothers who suffer the loss of a child through miscarriage or have a stillborn baby need support from friends and family. Remembering the experience with them and allowing them to speak about their loss is crucial for acceptance and healing.

Our friendship was put to the test that year. We each had to deal with motherhood in a different way and somehow carry on with life even though things would never be the same. Our memories of pre-motherhood were filled with laughter and fun times. We did everything together and there were no secrets. We survived the adversities and now we have a special relationship. We are there for each other no matter how much time passes or the miles between us. We always seem to pick up where we leave off.

I walked a fine balance the rest of my pregnancy. I appeared to be happy and joyful on the outside but in the back of my mind I feared that my baby would die or be deformed physically or mentally. I decided that it was my fate and that was only fair, because I was still blessed with a baby in my tummy. I also hid my joy from Kathy, not wanting to hurt her. She tried to make me feel comfortable around her and asked about the baby's kicks, the clothes, and the nursery. She bought me toy animals for the baby's room and gave me her maternity clothes. Kathy even came with me when I went for my ultrasound. Looking back on the last four months of my pregnancy, I was depressed and saddened by what happened to my friend Kathy. Research has shown that depression from experiencing traumatic events during pregnancy can contribute to PPD.[3]

The weekend before my due date, protein was found in my urine. It was very disconcerting. My doctor sent me to Medicine Hat, the city where I was to give birth, for a twenty-four hour urine analysis. I was a little scared and phoned my mother. As any concerned parents would be, mine immediately drove to the hospital to be with me. My urine test turned out fine and at 10:00 pm Saturday evening I started having my first contractions. I was so excited and wanted to get labour moving, so Curtis and I walked through hallways and up and down many stairs. We timed the contractions but they were far apart and not terribly painful. The nurses informed me that I would not be having a baby that evening. One of the nurses gave me a shot of Morphine that helped me to sleep. I had a great sleep which was good, because much rest was needed for the exhausting and traumatic events that were to occur.

I woke up on Sunday feeling refreshed and fine. The contractions had subsided. My parents arrived and we ate breakfast together. My contractions slowly started again. The breakfast did not agree with me and I vomited in the hospital bathroom. My parents and I decided to go to the mall even though I was still a little shaky. In retrospect I am not sure this was a good idea but I do love to shop! We decided to separate at the mall. I went with my mom and the men went on their own. We were there about an hour when my contractions started to get painful and I was having trouble walking. My mother took me back to the hospital. She dropped me off and then went to find Curtis. When he arrived, I hugged him and began to rock back and forth with every contraction which seemed to help with the pains. I was not offered an epidural, or any pain medication. The rest of the day was a blur.

I started to feel the urge to push around 9:00 in the evening. The nurses checked me and I was dilated seven centimeters. The toughest struggle of my life was about to begin. Two kindly nurses worked with Curtis and I for the next few hours. Because I was so far dilated, I wasn't able to receive any pain medication but I was able to have Nitrous Oxide (laughing gas). I felt sick to my stomach after breathing some of the gas. The nurses encouraged me to try again to help breathe through my contractions. Eventually I gave in to the pain and it seemed to help tremendously. The doctor broke my water which was a great relief. I pushed for two hours, but I think I lost track of time. Finally Cameron's head crowned. The doctor asked Curtis and I if it was alright to give me an episiotomy. We agreed. I was numb from the needle but didn't get cut after all, because I felt the urge to push one last time, and I delivered our little boy.

There were many people in the room. Cameron was placed on my belly. He was the most beautiful boy I had ever seen! The first thing I noticed about him was his very long fingers. They reminded me of my father. Cameron was taken away from me for a series of regular tests. I was so excited! I remember saying to Curtis that, "We did it!" We got through it together! I was so proud of myself! I didn't scream or even swear during the event! The student doctor began to massage my tummy to remove the placenta and then she asked me to give a little push. The placenta slid out with little effort. Cameron was given to me to hold. He was all bundled up. We took pictures with the doctor. I felt elated! I was "higher than a kite!" Curtis held Cameron when I was stitched. Unfortunately, I was told I had a third degree tear. The procedure started to hurt so severely that I grabbed the laughing gas. The room began to spin. I felt like I was on a Ferris Wheel and being stitched at the same time! I remember that it was the worst part of the whole experience!

My parents waited patiently to see their first grandchild. They came into the birthing room. They were Cameron's first visitors and they were so excited. It had been a long day and we all needed rest. The nurses took Cameron away because it was one o'clock in the morning and everyone was exhausted. Curtis was to sleep on a recliner in the birthing room with me, but he decided this would be uncomfortable so he slept on the floor. A nurse came in, gave me a sponge bath and then urged me to urinate, but I could barely walk the six steps to the bathroom. Every muscle in my body ached. I eventually was able to squat. I couldn't pass urine but the nurse had a trick up her sleeve. She turned on the water tap and let it run for a few minutes. Slowly, the relief I had been aching for came. I used this method for the next few days. The nurse helped me back on the uncomfortable bed and turned the lights off so I could catch up on some much needed sleep. My body had to calm down, both mentally and physically, from the high feeling after the shock of giving birth. I was exhausted, but I had trouble relaxing. I was wondering about Cameron and how he was doing. I was also freezing cold and asked the nurses for more blankets. I eventually fell asleep, but only for a few hours.

The nurses came in at about 3:00 in the morning so that Cameron could nurse for the first time. I was eager to start breastfeeding. I knew that this was an important step for baby's growth and development. I began to breastfeed Cameron, but the nurses noticed that he was cold. I was naturally concerned and the nurse decided to get him under the heat lamps. Curtis ran back to the nursery and made sure everything was alright. We both tried to sleep for the next few hours.

The nurses woke me again around 7:00 in the morning and wheeled me to the maternity ward. I was given a private room which was really lucky. They gave me Cameron. We began the process of trying to breastfeed again. After giving birth, there seemed very little that you are embarrassed about. A few of the nurses positioned my breasts so that he could suck. He had a hard time latching on and we found out later that he was tongue-tied. He was unable to stretch his tongue out far enough to properly cup my nipple while nursing.

My parents and Kathy and Trent visited that morning. I knew that it would be difficult for them because they lost their baby, but I also knew they wanted to share this happy event with us. The day went by quickly as we marveled at our tiny gift. We kept a diary of the diaper changes and feedings. The nurses taught us how to burp and swaddle him. He rarely cried. We phoned family and friends to share our good news. Cameron was very special because he was the first grandchild for both our families.

The evening finally came and Curtis left the hospital around 10:00 pm to stay overnight at a friend's house. Cameron slept at the nurse's station throughout the night but was given to me for feedings. The nurses woke me around midnight for my first feeding. Things seemed to work well and Cameron was taken back to the nurse's station when we were done. About five hours later, I awoke crying and screaming in a cold sweat. I had a nightmare that the nurses gave Cameron to me bloody and dead! I couldn't shake the intense horror of the dream! I hurried to the nurse's station and asked if I could take a peek at him. Cameron was bundled up, and sleeping like an Angel.

I still felt nervous and wanted to talk to someone for comfort. I did not want to wake Curtis knowing that he needed a good night's sleep. I decided to call my mother. It was still quite early and my sister Deana answered, half asleep and disorientated. She didn't expect to hear me crying. I asked to speak to mom but she said she had already left for work. My sister tried to calm me down. Uncannily enough, when I explained to her what was happening she wondered whether I had the symptoms of Postpartum Depression.

I went back to my room still feeling shaken and decided to call the nurses. I did not want to be alone. A nurse came and asked me what was wrong so I told her about the nightmare. She patted my back and reassured me that Cameron was okay. I felt a little better and tried to go to sleep. I awoke a couple of hours later and called Curtis to come as soon as possible. The nurses brought Cameron in for me to breast feed. I was visited by the on-staff doctor. He asked how I was feeling and inquired about the dream. I recalled the dream and how much it had upset me. They were obviously worried about what would have caused such a nightmare and looking for any other symptoms.

The next day was a blur! There were feedings, diaper changes, forms to fill out, nursing procedures and lactation consultations. I wanted to be successful at feeding Cameron but I was having a terrible time getting him to suck. My breasts were extremely sore and I cringed when his nails scratched my skin! I suffered terrible after pains that felt as bad as labour contractions. I was given extra strength pain killers and more pills to help me have a bowel movement. I was avoiding going to the bathroom because I feared that my insides would fall out.

The morning went by quickly and after lunch Cameron drifted to sleep in my arms. Curtis stepped out to get us coffee. I held Cameron and stared out the window. After having very little sleep during the last forty-eight hours, I found that my mood was no longer elated. I was starting to feel gloomy and there was the presence of a nervous stomach that I hadn't had since high school. As I glanced out the window people were coming and going. There were lots of trees and apartment buildings near the hospital. Cameron snored soundly. The window was open. I could hear the birds chirping while I sat there silently listening to the chatter of visitors. I began to day-dream. Maybe I was half asleep. All of a sudden, I heard a voice in my head say, "Smother." Why would I say that? There it was again; "Smother," again and again; "Smother, smother, smother, smother." I was scared and shaking. I also began to see frightening images in my head; images too difficult to talk about. All I could do was shake my head in an effort to make them go away.

I came back to reality when I heard footsteps, but I was sickened by myself. Why was I thinking those evil thoughts? I loved my new son with all my heart. What was wrong with my head? Curtis wasn't gone long but it seemed like an eternity. He walked in and whispered, "Hello," not wanting to wake Cameron. I tried to hide the panicked look on my face as I smiled and whispered, "Hello," back and took my coffee. In that instant my mask was born. I told Curtis I had to go to the bathroom. I closed the door and looked in the mirror. I could barely look at myself. I quietly spoke to the image in the mirror, "What the f… is wrong with you?" I wanted to vomit! I would never hurt Cameron! I told myself to stop over and over again. I wanted to run away, to scream, but the voice in my head wouldn't stop. I flushed the toilet and ran water in the sink. I wasn't crazy and this wasn't happening to me! I dismissed the voice and left the bathroom. That night I dreaded Curtis having to leave, but I tried to appear as if everything was fine. I was scared to be alone and didn't want to experience any more terrifying dreams. I also didn't want to be alone with the voice or the images that seemed to creep in my mind when I was trying to relax. I felt nervous and sick to my stomach. I was also dreading the next feeding!

It was two days since Cameron was born and I was growing increasingly anxious and scared. The voice was still popping up in my mind and I was aware that there was something seriously wrong with me. We began the morning nursing which was overwhelming, frustrating and painful. When Cameron tried to suck, I felt tears well up in my eyes. The student nurse tried to help. Curtis sat back patiently for the last few days as I tried to breastfeed our son with little success. Cameron desperately needed nourishment because he was beginning to have Jaundice. Finally, when my tears and Cameron's howls began to grow unbearable, Curtis demanded that the nurse bring us a bottle and someone who knew how to use it! I was relieved, but also felt very disappointed and guilty. Everywhere I turned there were signs that read "Breast is Best." I had also been lectured by my younger university-bound sister, Robin, on the importance of breastfeeding for a child's development. An older nurse arrived toting a bottle. She showed us how easy it was to use and explained the ingredients in the formula. Cameron started sucking immediately and we were so relieved.

Everyone in the room was happy except me. Even though Cameron ate well, I continued to cry. Curtis and the nurse inquired about my behaviour. I was afraid to admit what was wrong, but I couldn't take another day of being terrified. I explained that there was something horrible happening to me, and that I was hearing a voice in my mind and seeing terrifying images. The student nurse rubbed my back then she left the room to get the head nurse.

Curtis sat down and held Cameron. I'm sure by now that he was in shock. The nurse returned with a doctor and asked me to repeat what was happening. I told him, "There's something wrong with me, I keep hearing the voice in my head say, 'Smother'." The doctor sat there and listened to me. "I don't want to hurt Cameron, but the voice inside keeps saying 'Smother.' I don't know what to do? What is wrong with me?" The doctor said he thought that what I was experiencing was Postpartum Psychosis. We were silent; neither Curtis nor I had heard of this before. Yet apparently, Postpartum Psychosis can affect one in a thousand women. [4] The doctor recommended medication to treat my condition.

The nurses checked in every hour and I was evaluated by various doctors throughout the day. I was also assessed by a psychiatrist who prescribed an antidepressant and an anti-psychotic medication. The doctor suggested that I have regular naps during the day because I was extremely sleep deprived. The nurses were also instructed to provide the night time feeding to Cameron, so that I could catch up on my sleep. This was a Godsend and helped my condition. Curtis was able to stay with me in my room because going to sleep was my scariest time.

We came to the realization that we had a serious problem, and Curtis and I discussed ideas of what we would do when I was discharged. I needed someone to be with me because I was very fearful of being alone with Cameron. I called my mom later that evening and told her that things were not going well. I avoided telling her the whole truth. I casually mentioned that I was going to be given medications. My mom is a nurse, raised three daughters, and is a strong and independent person. Considering her knowledge and experience, her first reaction was to discourage me from taking any medications. I knew I had to tell her about everything I was experiencing. I divulged that I was hearing a voice in my head telling me to harm Cameron and seeing violent pictures. She was silent for a moment, and then agreed with the medications. Mom then told me that she loved me. I asked her if she could come and stay with me for a week. She said she had planned to anyway. I was unsure how long they would keep me in the hospital but I told her I would call her the following day.

We got into a routine over the next few days. I truly believe God only gives you what you can handle. Thankfully he gave us an angel baby. Cameron was truly sweet. He rarely cried and slept for hours at a time. Everything came easy as far as he was concerned. We certainly didn't need any further stress. Curtis never left me alone for very long. He stood nearby with the open bathroom door when I showered and got dressed. We all had regular naps during the day. The nurses administered pain and anti-anxiety medication to calm me down so that I could sleep. I took anti-depressants and anti-psychotic medication to stop that annoying voice in my head. This was the beginning of a sleeping cocktail that I would come to rely on and use to medically relax.

The voice in my mind stopped after the second day. I was so excited when I went for a shower that I could only hear the familiar songs I knew in my head. We nicknamed Cameron, "Mister Short Pants." I'm not sure why, maybe because he was so tiny. We were spoiled with kind, caring nurses who offered advice and who all doted on Cameron. I continued to have terrifying visions especially when settling down to sleep. I tried to be strong and not cry but, I was very sickened by the thoughts, and I was ashamed.

I phoned Kathy and she asked how things were going. People were wondering when I would be home because a normal hospital stay was usually only two days. I told her about the nightmare, the voice, and the visions. I said I would need her to support me now. We conspired to tell friends that I had been torn badly and needed healing and that Cameron had Jaundice, which wasn't a lie.

She promised to come and visit me on Friday. I trusted her with my darkest secret and she remained true to me.

Over the next few days we tried to remain calm and positive. The nurses were terrific, very helpful and sympathetic. Someone was always coming in to check on us, to check on Cameron or to hand out pills. Cameron went under the billy lights for his Jaundice, when he wasn't feeding. It bothered me that he was away so much, but I knew he was happy. He didn't seem to mind the lights at all.

Friday came and my family doctor from Oyen stopped in to see how his patient was doing. He must have heard about my condition because he knew what was going on. He said not to worry and that he had treated this before in South Africa. I would have weekly visits with him to report on my prognosis. He was a very kind man and I trusted him.

The Public Health nurse from Oyen was also in Medicine Hat and she stopped by to see me. She was aware of my problem and explained about a free home visitation program in Alberta where a health worker could visit me weekly. The worker happened to be my neighbor, and I really liked her funny demeanor. I was starting to feel that maybe I was going to be okay at home with this support system set in place. The medical staff did as much as they could, but they didn't share with me a few key things about my illness and the medications. I didn't know that I would feel like a zombie with little or no emotion; that I would not cry, but have no elation either, that I would be a walking, breathing, thinking, shell of a person; that the antipsychotic medication would make me hungry to the point of starving; that I would be tired all the time and gain weight rapidly. I didn't have the skill, knowledge, ability or self-esteem to ask questions about my illness or the medications. I was too overwhelmed and I just did what they told me to do as most patients do.

Special visitors also came to the hospital by the end of the week, Cameron's grandparents. We knew how lucky we were to have such loving grandparents on both sides of the family. Curtis's parents, Lynda and Bob, made the long trip from Moose Jaw and were so excited to hold Cameron and love him. When Curtis's mom held him she whispered into his ear and it was cute. They were both so excited to have a grandchild. When we told them about my illness, they were both very supportive. Curtis's dad made a point of telling him how good it was that I admitted that there was something wrong. I will never forget that! It was important to know that I had the courage to ask for help even in the beginning, and to not feel ashamed or hide my truth. Sometimes that is the only way one will get better!

Curtis's brother, Patrick, flew in from Ottawa as well. He was so excited to be an uncle. He made the trip back home with us to Oyen and cooked us a wonderful supper. I'll never forget the delicious meal, especially since we had been eating hospital food for a week. It was so nice to be home. Our family truly helped us out through everything and we were so very lucky to have their support. Patrick headed home the next day.

My mother arrived shortly thereafter, toting organization and lots of help. She got us on a system for bottle feeding and helped me get the house decorated for Christmas. She encouraged me to get out of the house and show Cameron to various friends. This kept me busy and I could forget about the intrusive thoughts. Mom was great and showed me that I could manage taking care of Cameron. She was there when I needed to cry. Sometimes I just broke down when Cameron was asleep and she hugged me and told me it would be okay.

The first week ended quickly. We had a few visitors and received many gifts. Everyone in town welcomed new babies. It was a joyous event. Everything looked peaceful on the outside; a new mother and an angelic baby. I wasn't okay though. I was sickened by the visions and worried about what would happen when the time came to be on my own. I knew I wouldn't harm Cameron, but what about my sanity?

Curtis's mother arrived by bus almost as my mother walked out the door. She was also a great help. She was very kind and always made me feel comfortable.

She loved to give Cameron a bath and showed me a way to give him a sponge bath. When Curtis and I gave him a bath before he had always cried, this bothered me because I hated to hear him cry and bath time was difficult with my visions. She placed all his baby items and clothes on the dining room table beside a tub of warm water. She then undressed him and wiped his whole body starting with his face. She sang songs to Cameron and he seemed to love this new bath. Lastly, she placed him in the small tub and splashed water on his bottom. She then put lotion on him. He smelled so sweet! I took this practice over and began to be less afraid of bath time.

It felt good to have someone around during the day. When I was busy, the visions were less frequent and I didn't notice them as much. The week was ending and I was petrified about taking care of Cameron on my own. Just before leaving the hospital I was advised by a health professional that I shouldn't tell others of my postpartum illness because most people did not understand it, and that I would likely be alienated. I did not know how I was going to keep this a secret from my friends, especially when I needed help. There was hope though because I was not totally alone. Another friend of mine, Sherry, had also given birth to a little girl a month earlier. We planned to keep busy going for walks and getting together.

The day Curtis's mom left, I visited Sherry. I kept the secret from her for eight months after coming home with Cameron. I know now that she helped me get through the loneliness and isolation I felt as a new mother without family around.

On that first day alone with Cameron, the hardest thing I found was coming home to an empty house, putting Cameron to bed and believing that I would not harm him. The panic and anxiety I felt that day was overwhelming, but I made it through the couple of hours on my own before Curtis came home from work. I was okay. Luckily, Cameron took to a routine instantly. Caring for him was very easy, and thankfully so. If he had been colicky or overly fussy, I don't know what I would have done. As it was, it took all my strength to battle with the visions throughout each day. This was very frustrating and scary! I had no mother close by to come to my aide when I needed to cry, or scream, or just take a break. I was the sole caregiver to my son during the day. My husband was a tremendous help in the evenings and weekends. However, over the next eight months, I endured a roller coaster of depression. The drugs made me sleepy, tired and ravenously hungry. The weight that was supposed to melt off wasn't. I was gaining even more. I had very little energy but somehow the laundry and house cleaning and daily chores got done. I lost interest in everything that I had enjoyed doing before Cameron was born. I found keeping the house clean and taking care of my son was enough strain just to get through the day.

All new mothers experience the stress of taking care of a little human being, like bottles, bathing, feeding and washing clothes. What a mother usually does not experience are thoughts of harming her little one; those frightening, intruding, disturbing thoughts, and the sick feeling of guilt and shame that comes after experiencing them. My doctor wanted me to track them, but at first there were too many in a day. Things were bad. I became obsessed with the visions. There were thoughts of smothering, drowning and on and on they went ... I don't know if anyone who reads this story will realize just how bad they were or what I was experiencing for those eight months. I won't go into graphic detail about the visions because those are negative thoughts and I don't want to relive them. Also, I am mindful of mothers who are currently suffering from "visions," and I do not want them to create any more sickening thoughts from reading my descriptions.

We were home for less than a few weeks when Cameron was waking up around four in the morning for his feedings. I would get up and warm a bottle and go down stairs to watch television. I was so sick and overwhelmed with visions and obsessions, that after I was done feeding Cameron and brought him back to our room (he slept in a bassinet in our room for three months), I would wake Curtis up so that he could check to see if Cameron was still breathing. I did this so that Curtis knew that I hadn't harmed our son while he was sleeping. I was also worried and obsessed about Sudden Infant Death Syndrome (SIDS).

If it should happen to Cameron, I would likely be blamed because of my illness! Looking back I think that best describes the "Hell on Earth" that we lived through. Curtis understood this need and checked Cameron every night!

I kept up the charade for eight months ... eight months of secret suffering! I wore the mask and hid my shameful truth! People thought I was a great new mother and that I had everything under control, but I didn't. I had thoughts of doing terrible things to my son. I didn't think them up. I was not evil. The thoughts would just pop into my head as simply as thinking you need a glass of water or something to eat. The pills never took the thoughts away. Some days I wondered why I was even on the medications, but I kept popping them faithfully every morning and every night.

My marriage took a beating. I am sure my husband experienced post-traumatic stress disorder. Every day he left for work wondering if he would find us both dead when he came home. Just imagine how you would feel leaving your spouse knowing that she was having those thoughts, and what the statistics were of it ending in tragedy. We hear in the news about the tragic endings. Sometimes these stories crept up on me unexpectedly. Like one day while sitting in the tub reading a People magazine, I opened to the article about a mother who drowned her five children in the bath tub. This mother suffered from Postpartum Psychosis. I sat there reading it and crying because I knew that it could have been me they were talking about! That story affected me deeply and I avoided reading it again. Somehow I knew I would survive and not be the centre of such a tragedy.

We flew to Ottawa, when Cameron was eight months old, to visit Curtis's brother for two weeks. I was exhausted all the time and Cameron wasn't sleeping well. Although it was supposed to be a happy family vacation, I was still depressed and the visions continued to plague me when I was alone. I became more depressed because I gained weight. Curtis and I also had little or no personal time together for nearly eight months. We made a date to go to a museum to have a few hours to ourselves. The time we spent alone was fun.

We went to the O'Reilly reunion at Curtis's aunt's farm. The O'Reilly's were a great bunch and loved Cameron the instant they met him. I don't know how I seemed to outsiders, maybe normal enough. Yet Curtis's brother's friend, Fraser, came over for supper and noticed that something was wrong. Curtis mentioned this to me later. The truth is that I knew the medications were not working. The voices were gone but I was still having lots of visions of harming Cameron. There were too many to count and they just popped in my mind and terrified me. I started to wonder if I was crazy enough to think those thoughts, was I crazy enough to do those unimaginable things. They say, "The eyes are a window to the soul." If you looked through my eyes and truly saw what I saw, then you could understand the sadness, fear and pain I experienced those eight months.

We arrived home from Ottawa and then two days later headed to Sundre, a small Alberta town, for my family reunion. It was definitely a whirlwind trip but I was excited to see my aunts, uncles and cousins. In the evening, almost everyone went to the rodeo while my Aunt Karen and I opted to stay home. My aunt asked how I was coping with motherhood and whether I had experienced any depression. She listened with acceptance and understanding while I tearfully described my symptoms. She really helped me by sharing some of her struggles with motherhood. I have felt a strong bond with her since then. I often recall that night when I shared my ugly secret! I felt she really reached out to me and it validated my feelings. Sometimes the best way to help a woman suffering with PPD is to let her know that she is not the only one. Everyone feels down at one time or another in their life and we all need to be accepted.

I realized how exhausted I was when we drove home, from the lack of sleep, too much excitement and all the late nights. I was busy and surrounded by family for about three weeks. It distracted me from my thoughts for the most part. However, the loneliness and realization that I had a huge problem, one that wasn't being helped by medication, was terrifying me even more. The next day was a regular day. Curtis left for work and I awoke. I was very tired and wanted to sleep more. I felt disgusted with my body and with myself. I was back home into the old routine. I was alone for eight hours filled with obsessive visions. Everything triggered the visions. I had terrifying thoughts at routine times like when carrying a cup of hot coffee or walking down the stairs to the basement. I also had fears about using plastic bags, knives, bleach, bathtubs, and pillows. The kitchen was an unfriendly place for me and I hid everything. The old adage, "out of sight out of mind," was very true during my illness. These terrible thoughts brought unbearable levels of anxiety. If you have never had an anxiety attack, it feels more severe than when you are a child writing an exam and realizing that you forgot to study, or getting ready to play a sport and you're very nervous about it, or public speaking in front of a large audience. I'm referring to the anxiety that makes you nauseous and sweaty. I was having many of these frightening attacks each day. The attack that day was worse than usual. I was nervous, overwhelmed and scared. I couldn't catch my breath or think straight.

It was about 12:45 pm and I knew Curtis would be home at one o'clock for lunch. All mothers, even those without PPD, count-down anticipating the time their spouse will walk through the door and relieve them. Fifteen minutes seems like fifteen hours when you are having an anxiety attack and visions. Cameron and I snuggled on our bed. I looked up and saw the ceiling fan. I realized how it could be dangerous as well. As it twirled around and around I thought of how it could hurt someone. I was so scared because it was quiet in the house, and I was so alone with these thoughts. I wanted to scream! I picked up Cameron and started pacing back and forth down the hallway. I was quickly losing control. "This is enough!" I wanted to scream. "Enough! Enough! Enough! Why is this happening to me and why has nobody helped me!" I felt so angry and desperate! I was living in "Hell on Earth" inside my head! Sickening thoughts, scary thoughts! I just could not take it anymore! I was pushed past my breaking point! I wanted to kill myself and end the nightmare! The mask had to come off!

I could not bear it anymore. My doctor told me that if it ever got to be too much, I should immediately go to the hospital. He would help. Curtis came home and saw that I was crying and clearly distraught. I told him that I couldn't take it anymore and needed help. We called Kathy to look after Cameron and phoned the hospital to notify the doctor. I decided right then and there that I would no longer keep the secret from my friends and family. Everyone would know what was going on. That was the only way I would get help. I decided that I didn't care anymore who knew. From then on the shame left me.

Curtis drove me to the hospital. I was crying as I walked through the emergency doors. I am sure that the staff were stunned by my admissions that day, but they listened to my story and tried to understand my feelings and symptoms. My doctor arrived very quickly and I was admitted. I revealed, with brutal honesty, that I couldn't manage the visions on my own anymore or keep the secret. I just wanted to see a specialist and get treated. I spent the rest of the afternoon feeling relieved but also scared because I didn't know what was going to happen to me.

Curtis followed my wishes and began to phone family and friends and let them know what had been going on. He called Troy and Sherry first. We had been friends for three years and had so much in common. Curtis and Troy were volunteer firemen. I pretty much spent every day with Sherry for the past eight months. I never disclosed that I was dealing with something so terrible. I remember that day when I was admitted into the hospital very clearly. Later in the afternoon while sitting in my room resting, Sherry came to see me. With tears in my eyes I looked into hers and said, "Now you know the truth." I realized that true friends accept your flaws and stand by you in your darkest hours.

Another friend, Wendy, whom I did not share my secret, was also pregnant at the same time I was. Wendy's husband and Curtis worked together. Our children were born only days apart. We would get together weekly for coffee and swap stories about the newborns. I remember her coming to visit one time and panicking because she had forgotten gripe-water to calm her daughter's colic. Noticing Cameron's calm demeanor, she looked me square in the face and commented on how I probably didn't even own any nor need it. I thank God that I was blessed with a calm baby, who rarely cried, especially with my illness. I never told Wendy about my situation. When we discussed it years later, she said she sensed that something wasn't quite right. She just couldn't put her finger on it. Wendy remembered getting the call about my illness and the feeling of being "hit by a train." She had no idea what we had been dealing with for eight months and was beside herself with emotion and worry.

The doctor decided to send me to a larger hospital where they could do a more thorough assessment and provide treatment. I packed my bags and was ready to leave. This was a very sad day because I left my son and husband behind, and took a three-hour ambulance trip to the hospital. I looked terrible but I thought that I might as well be comfortable and dress in my favourite leisure suit. I was hoping that I looked like a typical mental-health patient. This wasn't a fashion show though and after all that I had been through, my appearance was the last thing on my mind. I hugged and kissed my son one last time and was carried by stretcher to the ambulance. The ambulance drivers were very professional and made me feel comfortable. I could not relax, which I guess would be expected just knowing that I was heading to the "loony bin." I silently laid on that stretcher for the three-hour drive. When we arrived, they escorted me to the ward and made sure that I was admitted. I felt nervous, alone, scared and relieved all at once. Those three weeks in the Calgary Foothills Hospital Mental Health Ward were three weeks of my life that I will never forget!

I told myself that I was in the Psychiatric Ward because I was a horrible mother who had thoughts about harming her son. The real truth was that I had courageously admitted that I had a problem and asked for help to deal with it. It is so easy to beat yourself up. I had to stop the internal warfare. By this time, I didn't worry anymore about how things would appear to outsiders. I think you get over that when you realize things aren't black and white. This happened when I became knowledgeable about mental illness and Postpartum Depression. I realized that I was not alone and was told that many women experience PPD and many more that probably do not report their symptoms.

I couldn't believe that I was really in the Mental Health Ward. I saw Electroconvulsive Shock Therapy (ECT) in the movie "One Flew Over the Cuckoos' Nest." My mother warned my husband that I might need ECT and that it wasn't as inhumane as it used to be. I told Curtis that I was going to pretend that I was going to the spa and tried to imagine a better place. Being the logical man that he is, he suggested that I should not pretend anymore, and that I should just face reality and get help.

The food was horrible! There were so many things to get used to. It was like the first day of school when you don't know a soul and you're so alone. Luckily the Mental Health Ward I had been sent to was very relaxed. People with more severe mental health disorders were admitted to a higher security ward. I was somewhat comfortable and relieved. Many patients were coping with alcohol addictions, anorexia or depression. The other patients didn't seem to get too excited about anything. They were friendly and welcomed me. I was able to get lots of sleep but of course I was still really tired in the morning because it was a drugged induced sleep.

One of the ways I survived the first eight months on the medications was to drink really strong coffee. Every evening I would order coffee for breakfast and every morning there was my breakfast but no coffee. Was I really going crazy or was someone messing with me and stealing my coffee? So I ran down the stairs to the main entry way and grabbed a coffee from Starbucks. This stuff was amazing! It woke me up! To this day I still have a love affair with Starbucks coffee. I am literally a zombie until I have had my first cup. After a few days, I finally got annoyed and asked the nurse if someone was taking my coffee. She laughed and said that they didn't serve coffee in the Mental Health Ward because it had caffeine in it and caffeine was a drug. Go figure, all these drugged people and nothing to wake them up in the morning!

I was there only a couple of days and realized that I better find a few more friends or this was going to be a very lonely place. Talking to the other patients helped pass the time. During the day, I would sit outside with the smokers, usually the most interesting people, and listen to them talk about their lives. They had great stories that would make me laugh and forget about why I was there. As far as they knew, I was there for Postpartum Depression. I would leave out the extreme details of my condition and was careful who I shared my story with because I did not want to be judged by strangers.

I noticed a new girl in the ward one day walking around wearing a hospital nightgown. I never got one of these nightgowns, but she had to wear hers. She looked really angry at the nurses. She was confined to the ward and not allowed to "escape" and go outside with the rest of the group. I sat beside her the next day at breakfast. We made small talk and I introduced myself. I never knew the extent of her symptoms, but I figured it had something to do with depression. We found it easy to talk with one another and spent the next few days getting acquainted. We spent a lot of time together during the following three weeks going to therapy sessions, craft sessions and workout sessions. In the last few days before I was scheduled to come home, I began to cry. I missed Cameron so much and couldn't stand it anymore. My new friend held me and told me it would be okay. She reassured me that we were almost free! She needed to complete the Outpatient Program and I was going home. I was going back to reality. I miss her and I am forever grateful for her friendship during my stay. I hope that she will read this and someday we will connect again. She helped me get through those three lonely weeks.

I was allowed to go on day and weekend passes because my hospital stay was a lengthy one. Curtis drove the three-hour drive with Cameron to visit me on most weekends. We even stayed in a hotel together one weekend. Curtis always stood by and supported me. He traveled a lot, he slept very little and he worried constantly. He somehow managed to work and hold down a very stressful job. Curtis was literally a single parent under excessive stress for those three weeks. How he didn't give up or have a nervous breakdown himself was amazing!

Our families helped us tremendously while I was hospitalized by caring for Cameron when Curtis would make the trips between Oyen, Moose Jaw and Calgary to drop him off and pick him up. They couldn't look after Cameron for the entire three weeks so we had to find a baby-sitter. One of our friends, Erica, who was a teacher, offered to look after Cameron for the last two weeks of my hospital stay. She really helped us out of a bind and I will admit I never worried about Cameron while he was in her care. It gave me peace of mind knowing that he was with such a kind person, while I was off getting my head together.

I had a few visitors that really helped validate that I was doing the right thing to ask for help and that I shouldn't be ashamed. Two of my friends actually lived in the same city as the hospital. My friend Terri took me out for supper when I got an evening pass. She listened to my story and offered words of encouragement. Although we had not seen much of each other over the last few years, we were able to talk freely and comfortably. I felt at ease sharing my secret with her. I knew she had her own struggles and that she understood what it was like to be searching for happiness. She offered her house as a place for Curtis to stay while I was in the hospital.

My high school friend, Pam, also rescued me one afternoon from the mundane of the hospital so that we could go shopping. I forgot what I was really in this city for, even if just for awhile. We made an appointment to get my hair cut at a fancy salon. I needed time free from the visions, free to laugh, free to forget that I was away from my eight-month old son for the very first time. It was an afternoon of giggling like school girls and gossiping about old times. We still keep in touch no matter how busy we are, and I will always have a bond with her because I have known her for so long. We can share a laugh and both know that we can be our true selves with each other. My friends supported me throughout my battle and helped me to accept myself. I was surrounded by a community of women and without their help I would not have survived.

When I was in the hospital, the psychiatrist asked if I would speak about my illness to a group of students. He was also going to ask questions about my history of depression during the talk. I agreed to this because I thought it would help the students understand my illness. We met in a small room that had a two-way mirror. I understood that there were people behind the glass, watching me and listening to my story because I watched enough crime movies. I felt that I could talk freely, without judgment because they were educated about mental illness unlike the general public and I couldn't see their faces. I was still a little scared and nervous, but my doctor did a good job of making me feel comfortable. I quickly relaxed and described my condition and shared my life story.

It was difficult to admit to others that I was in a Psychiatric Ward. It was unbearable at first to admit to myself that I was actually there. I can laugh now, four years later. It was like prison in some respects. There were no gang beatings and you did get passes for good behaviour. There were visits with the psychologist who suggested I think of a purple elephant whenever I had a vision. Another strategy was to snap a rubber band on your wrist to chase away the thoughts. My visions were so plentiful that my arm was purple from the constant snapping. Everyone wondered why I thought a rubber band was fashionable as a bracelet! Curtis suggested we get a shirt made that said "My wife went to the Psych Ward and all she brought me back was this crappy T-shirt." We tried to make light of a very sad and scary situation.

We went on an outing to the Calgary Zoo near the end of my stay. The heat was sweltering. There were ten patients and two staff members. On our way out of the van, as a joke, I yelled that everyone should scatter. "They will never be able to take us alive," I exclaimed. Although I was severely depressed, I still had a sense of humor. To celebrate my last night I got the group together and suggested that we have a pizza party. A few patients were surprised and thought that we wouldn't be allowed. They wondered what would be done with the hospital food. I didn't care and said that we would just let it sit there and send it back! It was funny. I think they thought I was crazy to make the suggestion, but I didn't care. The pizza party was great! We even finished the night with a movie, "The Pirates of the Caribbean." I had to do something to forget the pain in my stomach and the emptiness I felt when I thought about the reason I was here.

When the doctor informed me that I was ready to be released, I was so excited and couldn't wait to enjoy my son and all the comforts of home. I spent three weeks meditating, talking to counsellors, taking more medications, reading, walking, talking, learning about stress, doing puzzles and crafts, and meeting strangers with similar problems. I wouldn't say that I was cured because I wasn't, but I knew I wanted to be with my son and that I had the strength to go on with my life, visions or no visions. I also knew that I would need breaks away from my son in order to deal with the visions. This would be an issue to work on when I got home.

I had to prove that I was in touch with reality before I got my golden pass to leave. They actually had a test for this. It was actually quite a funny test. I had to make spaghetti, warm up canned vegetables in the microwave, count money, know the day, month, year, and how much money we had in the bank and what our mortgage and monthly bills were. I passed everything but embarrassingly enough, being married to a banker, I didn't really concern myself with our finances, so I guessed.

When I arrived home, I knew I would need to get out of the house and talk to people about my illness and tell them when I was having good days or bad days. I invited many of my friends over for coffee and talked freely about my illness. I kept myself busy and energized by walking and going out. Annie, the neighbour two houses down, was a sweet grandmother. She introduced herself and brought us a baby gift when Cameron was born. I promised her that I would stop by for coffee and bring Cameron for a visit. I have no doubt that she was really an Angel in disguise. Annie welcomed us to her home once a week. All I needed to do was call and tell her that I was having a rough day and she would invite me to her house. Her love for Cameron was obvious. There were always a lot of toys for him. Annie knew the truth about my illness but she never made me feel uncomfortable about it. She understood motherhood. We laughed together as she told funny stories about her own children. What a relief it was to forget about the visions for a couple of hours. I'll never forget Annie's kind heartedness and how she helped me. Cameron enjoyed yet another Grandma, but this one was right in our own hometown.

The whole town now knew my secret. Our friends and the community at large came to our aide. They sent cards or stopped in to see us and shared their support in person. I felt free suddenly. I wasn't alone in this battle. I began to schedule breaks for myself and arranged for someone I trusted to watch Cameron at times during the day. One of the kind mothers in the community offered to look after Cameron once a week. Her two younger daughters loved to play with him. This helped me tremendously.

We moved to Regina in August of 2005, after being away for nearly six years in Alberta. I was excited to move closer to home and finally have more of the support from family that I most desperately needed. I was excited too because I had been referred to a new counsellor and was hoping that she could help me. The visions were still there, haunting my thoughts. Maybe this counsellor would have ideas that I had not tried yet. She listened and told me about a Postpartum Depression Support Group offered through the YMCA. I was extremely thrilled because I knew that a group of mothers, who dealt with the same things and shared their stories, would be good for me. Maybe there would even be a mother with Postpartum Psychosis or Postpartum Obsessive Compulsive Disorder.

I phoned the meeting coordinator, Sally Elliot, and spoke about my illness and mood. She thought that I would benefit from the group and invited me to the meeting that was held on Wednesdays at noon. I was working part-time as an Administrative Assistant with a flexible schedule. I asked to have my days off switched to Wednesdays and started to attend the regular meetings. I was very nervous the first time I attended. I found the room but there was no one in it so I walked back to the elevator. A very tall woman got off the elevator and smiled as she walked past me. I didn't know it yet but this lady would later become one of my very best friends. I walked back to the room and sat down. Others, including the tall woman that I had seen at the elevator, gradually joined the group. Then Sally came in, and introduced herself and asked how I was doing. I felt better already and relief washed over me. I soon realized that a support group helped me feel better mainly because of the commonality of shared experiences. I was very nervous but as soon as it was my turn to talk everyone listened and nodded in agreement as I spoke about my experience. We were all tearful that first hour and a half. It was obvious how we needed each other. It was the best therapy I had ever had and it was free!

Tania was the first woman I met in the group. She was the lady I had seen getting off the elevator. Tania introduced herself and wasn't shy or worried about what anyone thought. I could tell that right away. This is what I mostly liked about her. She mentioned immediately that she had suffered psychosis and that she was on an anti-psychotic medication that she didn't like because it made her fat. Flashing lights and sirens went off in my head. Here was someone who was experiencing the same symptoms as me and she was on a similar medication. No one believed me that this medication made you fat or hungry. I gained forty pounds with the pregnancy, plus another thirty after childbirth. I couldn't stand myself but I was too depressed to do something about it.

Tania had told me about her high risk and traumatic pregnancy. Her daughter was born prematurely. After giving birth, Tania became manic and was unable to sleep for days. She was also admitted to the Mental Health Ward in Regina and said it was very scary. She was great to talk to. When others in the group mentioned that they had trouble cleaning the house while depressed, Tania said that she simply didn't clean. It was liberating to hear someone who did what she wanted and didn't feel guilty about it or feel that she was failing. Let's face it, most mothers don't enjoy cleaning but we do it anyway because it's expected. When you're sick, just getting the strength to get out of bed in the morning is a chore in itself. Luckily, I didn't have too much trouble getting out of bed or keeping the house somewhat clean. It gave me something to do when I was bored.

Tania also experienced visions. She said that when the visions came to her, she would just tell herself, "That's nice Tania, now move on!" She didn't validate the thoughts or give them importance. She was very intelligent and recognized that she was just experiencing a problem with her brain and that the visions were a result of that. I began to learn that if I ever wanted to get better I would have to be more accepting of myself, and to not get so stressed out about the visions. Maybe I would have Obsessive Compulsive Disorder for the rest of my life. After four years, I guess I was able to accept that, but I would have to learn to deal with the visions and not feel sick and disgusted with myself.

The more meetings we went to, the more we became comfortable with each other. I was searching for some friends because I found moving to a bigger center very lonely. We decided to go for coffee after one of our meetings. My support group became a place where I could find grace to heal and strengthen my damaged persona. It was at these coffee dates where we really began to forge a true friendship. We would talk about all sorts of topics and nothing was off limits. We talked about our children, our struggles with marriage and finding a balance with our husbands. Now that we had shared our deepest secrets there were less tears and more laughter. I was a regular member of the group and attended the postpartum support sessions every week. Other women would frequently join us and their stories would bring fresh tears and nods as we listened intently. Everyone understood what each other was going through. That connection was the greatest thing about the group. I had strong feelings and a desire that I should help others with this illness. That's when I met Carrie.

Carrie was the first person I tried to help and we became close friends. She entered the meeting looking scared and nervous. She told us that her daughter was colicky, and how she was sleep deprived and having anxiety attacks. The first thing I suggested was to get some help from family and medication to stop the anxiety. She had not yet accepted that what she was experiencing was Postpartum Depression. It became very apparent after she listened to the group. I felt so touched by her story because I had been there myself two years earlier. After the meeting, on the way to our cars, I patted her shoulder and told her it would get better. We exchanged phone numbers and I told her to call me if she needed any help. Carrie called a few days later to vent her frustrations. I told her to be patient because as time went on, it would get easier. It helped me so much to help others and to gain some friendships with such strong bonds.

My journey with this illness has had its peaks and valleys. At one point in March of 2006, I became really sick and had visions of suicide and slitting my wrists in the bathtub. I was depressed because of my weight. I was depressed because of the visions. I was depressed because my husband had become a prisoner to my illness. Our family was basically paralyzed in distress! I found it hard to be alone with my son, cope with work stress and manage the household. I did do all those things, yet it wasn't enough. I was not a happy person and I had no dreams or goals. I reached out for help again and went to the Emergency Ward.

I was finally seen by a doctor after a whole afternoon of waiting. I told her about my illness and the thoughts of suicide. I was literally alone this time because my husband was home with our son. I began to feel sorry for myself. I think everyone around me was exhausted as well, and did not know what to do anymore. God was watching over me and brought me Tania. She literally tracked me down, first stopping at the Psychiatric Ward to see if I was there. She pushed herself through the elevator doors with tears streaming down her face. She didn't want to return to that place and remember the past. Tania spent time on the Psychiatric Ward dealing with her own postpartum illness. The pain and memory from her stay was still raw. Yet, like a true friend, she swallowed her fear and forged ahead searching for me! She needed to tell me that I was okay and that this was not the place for me. She knew that staying there would not solve my problems.

I was so relieved that I wanted to cry when she walked through the door of the Emergency Ward. I hugged her and we talked for the next hour. The doctor came in and said that I was okay to go home. She reassured me by saying that there were patients in more dire need than me, and that I had a good support system and a good head on my shoulders. The doctor then suggested more counselling to treat the visions. This incident helped me to recognize that I would have good days and bad days and sometimes the bad days could be really bad. I also knew though that I had a support system that believed in me. The most important thing I needed to learn was to believe in myself!

I met Tania for coffee one evening and she began talking about her dreams and goals. She talked about traveling and finances and how one day she was going to meet Oprah. Just being around her changed my outlook on life. I told her about writing my story and how it was my hope to have it published one day. We brainstormed about it and concluded that it would indeed be an inspiring book for families suffering with postpartum illnesses. I left feeling somewhat deflated because after talking to Tania I realized that I have never really dreamed about my life or set life goals. I just lived my life day-to-day and never imagined the future. I realized Tania was doing something right and I sought to find out just what it was. My real dream was to tell my story, to help other women who were suffering in silence. I knew that there could be others like me experiencing the visions. Someone that was battling the same demons and she didn't have support!

Carrie gave me the book "The Secret." [5] She told me to read it because it would open my eyes and change my life. I was a little apprehensive and didn't really believe in miracles, but I began to read. That night I had the most relaxing sleep ever. I woke up with an amazing realization. I could not only control my horrible thoughts, but if I believed in my dreams and practiced thinking positively, I could control my reactions to stress and external threats. I could also produce more positive things in my life just by thinking positively about them. I had control over my entire destiny! I had been allowing my negative fears to control my life and I had been wasting so much energy worrying about everything. It was a self-fulfilling prophecy! The more I practiced "The Secret," the more I became aware of my control over my own thoughts. I also attended a session on Angel therapy at the public library and learned that Angels are around to protect us and all we have to do is ask them for help. In this session I also learned that we have two types of thoughts, thoughts of fear and thoughts of love. My obsessions were indeed fear-based thoughts. I came to the conclusion that I could continue down the path of complete fear for the rest of my life, or I could allow myself the intense freedom of believing in my strengths and could also give hope to other mothers. In other words, focus on thoughts of love. Aha! I began to believe that if we wanted this book to materialize, we had to dream about it! We knew we needed to find a publisher and that's where I thought the dream would end. We were just regular women, not trained writers, but that never stopped Tania from believing. She excitedly phoned me one day. She said that she had bumped into a publisher at a fundraising event and had discussed our plans for a book about PPD. They exchanged email addresses and planned to meet to discuss the possibilities of a book project. I couldn't believe it! I had been so used to negative thinking. Even still, I was weary and didn't tell anyone because I did not want to risk looking like a fool. The publisher, Peggy Collins, had just co-published a bestselling book called "Never Give Up – Ted Jaleta's Inspiring Story."[6]

Tania set up a coffee date with Peggy and one Saturday we all got ready to pitch our stories. I was very nervous because I wanted this so badly. The meeting went great and I began to realize that Peggy was a very likeminded person. We had similar beliefs and she was interested in our stories. We left the meeting knowing that she was seriously considering the project. I was so excited! We hugged and cheered but I noticed that Tania was kind of quiet. She said in a simple straightforward manner that she knew this would happen. She had been practicing "The Secret" longer than I had and she had become quite confident because of it.

We made plans to meet for another coffee date. Tania asked Elita, one of her friends who had been secretly suffering from PPD, to join us this time. Elita was interested in writing her story as well. She jelled immediately with the group and was excited to meet women who understood what she was feeling. That was how our story began, just four women dreaming, believing that one day soon we would break the silence, heal the pain and destroy the smiling mask! It is difficult to reflect back on such a horrible past but speaking and writing about it has allowed me to let go of the pain and move forward to help others.

Even though I experienced the most debilitating form of Postpartum Depression, it's important to note that I always loved my son very deeply. I did everything in my power to ensure that he had a happy childhood. This is true for the majority of PPD sufferers and one of the many misunderstood elements about the disease. These mothers love their children just as much as any other mother. Cameron and I share a wonderful, meaningful loving relationship. When Cameron was born, he instantly became our sweet little prince. He was tiny, only six pound fourteen ounces and had the sweetest cowlick, even though there was only a skiff of hair on his head. Lullabies were regular events in our home. I sang him "Baby Beluga," a song from my childhood and "Hush Little Baby," a song I used to sing to my sister when she was a baby. I learned new ways to be comfortable giving him his morning bath and I would even read him a story about bathing. I would rock him to sleep everyday for his mid-morning nap and loved watching him sleep. He rarely cried and on Christmas Eve, when he was two months old, he slept through the night for his first time. He was a very contented baby and would naturally go with any of the relatives or friends. I loved being a mother and even now that he is four, I still love to snuggle and play with him. It brings me great joy to read to him because that is a gift I feel I can share.

Our beautiful relationship continues. What fun Cameron and I have as we dance to the song "I like to move it, move it." He loves to dance and perform for people. Cameron and I often laugh when I say, I love you, he will say I love you "two" and I say love you "three", he'll say love you "four" and so on right until "twenty." I'm not much into wrestling which seems to be the sport Curtis enjoys with Cameron, but I love to give piggy back rides through the house and pretend that I am a horsy. I am very overprotective almost to a fault. My illness contributed to this to some degree but I think perhaps it's a normal maternal instinct. At least that's what I tell myself. Having Cameron has taught me to be self-sacrificing because his welfare is the most important thing. It's critical to find ways to not hang out in the dumps and feel sorry for myself the way I used to. I learned to look after myself so that I could look after him. I am thankful for my son and the gift that he is.

Since the first few hours of my illness, there was shock, tears and disbelief from my husband. I had just given birth to a beautiful boy twenty-four hours before, and then I was hearing voices in my head and seeing visions of harming him. These truths damaged our very happiness for the next four years of our lives, even though these admissions were likely the first steps in getting better. We never expected anything like this to happen and were unaware that having a child could leave a woman so debilitated. However, we realized that we were not given enough education about the illness from the medical community. We were sent home to fend for ourselves, without many resources.

We were coping the best we could, and even though from an outsider's view we were falling apart, we battled the toughest fight of our lives united and together. My husband explained to me right from the beginning that this illness was like any other illness, "Just like me having asthma." He reassured me that it wasn't my fault, just something that happened to my brain after giving birth. I will never forget those comforting words.

I realize that this illness was not easy on my relationships, especially Curtis's and mine. We pledged "in sickness and in health" when we took our vows, not knowing what was to follow. Curtis begged me to bring his wife back when I was in my darkest hours and I replied with tears that I was trying my best to be a good mother and a good wife. The real "me" was lost somewhere in the mental illness. The depression grabbed a hold of my soul and the obsessions sickened me for four years. They tore at my inner self, the beautiful caring self that I once was. All I wanted was for the visions to stop. All I needed was that the visions would stop. I cannot speak for Curtis, but I know that our love relationship was affected by anger and resentment. A huge strain was placed on our relationship because of my illness. We were unable to save our marriage because of the extreme stress and pressure that resulted. We tried hard to stay together but realized that we had endured too much pain. Luckily, we remained together long enough to enjoy our son's growth through his early childhood and will hold on to the memories forever of his birth, first words, and strong independency. Together we raised a child with kindness, intelligence and an enormous sense of humor. We cared so much for Cameron that we believed his emotional welfare was the most important. We both know that our love created him and together we will guide him through life.

I have managed to create a positive outlook for my future through much self reflection and struggle. Not only have my scars from this illness healed, but I feel I am an even better person than the person I was before my son was born. I am a more accepting, caring and positive person. Through my trials and knock downs, I always got back up. I will admit that throughout this four year ordeal, there were times when I contemplated suicide and believed those close to me would be better off without me. However, as my mother once "drilled" into my brain after an argument, "Suicide is the ultimate act of selfishness." She went on to say, "You are a mother and you owe it to yourself and your family to pull through and fight this fight."

The year 2007 marked my thirtieth birthday, and I decided after years of being a people pleaser, that I was going to start standing up for myself! My twenties were happy years but I was still a baby. I had no stretch marks or appearances of aging. My world changed forever when I had my son. I somehow managed to care for him although I was depressed, saddened and scared. He taught me what I've always known, that is, that I love children and their gifts. I love their beautiful smiles, snuggles, first words and their potential. With just a little TLC, children will blossom and grow. My friend Kathy told me that she didn't believe that women should worry too much about wrinkles, that if we didn't have wrinkles we have never really lived, we have never laughed and we have never cried. Our facial lines show the storms we've weathered and the joys we've experienced. Women should embrace their scars and wounds, and wrinkles with love for themselves.

I learned an important lesson from my illness. In order for mothers to fully appreciate their children, they periodically need a break from them. We can lose so much of our own identity in the first year of motherhood. We are becoming mothers, but our old selves are put out into limbo. Sometimes we don't have time to even brush our teeth or take a shower. Becoming a caregiver for a little being is sometimes very difficult. We can obviously get used to it, but when women have time for themselves, they become better mothers overall. This was especially apparent for me when my husband would give up his free time so that I could have a bath, go for a walk, go grocery shopping, or go for a massage. Time away meant time without the visions. It helped me walk that fine line of being able to cope instead of choosing suicide.

I believe that the initial first step of admitting that I had a problem and asking for medical help was what saved me. Going to the hospital on that grim day when I could not bear it any longer saved my life. I believe that finding a Postpartum Depression support group gave me the best coping skills and helped me to heal at a deeper level. Feeling validation from others and that I wasn't the only one dealing with this illness was also very important. The friends I made at the support group guided me to new ways of thinking about life and eventually encouraged me to be a survivor and not a victim. We were united together and we realized our full potential. We survived by using many tools and skills, and it is now our mission to spread the word and give hope to other women and families that are suffering. I have now accepted my illness as a gift that will create awareness and give hope to other people living in this inner "Hell." Women need to ask for help, to find a support group or start a support group, to stop blaming themselves, and stop being a victim to this illness. Being a mother and creating life is the most important thing in the world. We are creating the children of the future. We need to take hold of our power, and remember our strengths.

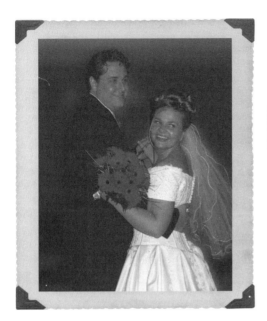

Elita's wedding photo

Elita after giving birth

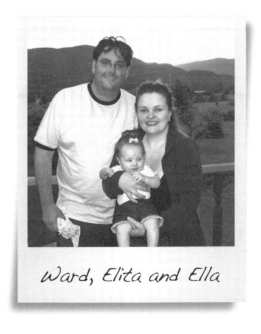

Ward, Elita and Ella

Chapter Two
Elita's Truth

You are today where your thoughts have brought you;
you will be tomorrow where your thoughts take you.
~ James Allen

My name is Elita Paterson. My husband Ward and I began our baby-making in 2004 with a miscarriage. I haven't been the same since.

My low self-esteem and anxieties especially came to light when the Pre-Natal Nurse, Sally Elliot, from the YMCA told me that I wasn't simply dealing with grief after my miscarriage, but that I was dealing with a much larger problem. All I felt was a looming sense of failure. She asked if I would consider this loss as a gift to myself, one that would help me to deal with my negative feelings, before we brought another baby into our lives. I struggled with depression and extreme anxiety most of my life and it was starting to control me.

It took another bout of depression before I would take her advice to heart. It was bad and I knew that I had to do something to change the way my life was going. I pursued some training and completed a nine-week intensive personal growth program, with amazing results. I followed the philosophy of the program the next five months, "creative self-management through the understanding of energy dynamics." It was life changing. I became conscious about what I ate, meditated every day, and applied the healing tools that I had learned to increase my awareness. I progressively stopped consuming sugar, caffeine, alcohol, wheat and meat. I became involved in yoga and walked regularly. I was dropping inches and feeling energetic after the first month and even more with each passing month. I was aware that I was taking back my power. I had a renewed faith in myself and in the Universe/God/my Higher Spirit, and realized that I could achieve whatever I believed. Everything was at my fingertips. All I had to do was focus on what I wanted like, a reliable car, a more meaningful relationship, a healthy baby etc. The program resonated with my constant desire to learn more about my purpose in life and myself.

I experienced tremendous growth and confidence during this time. "Voila!" I became pregnant in June 2006! I was so sick! I experienced nausea all day long beginning in my sixth week that continued well into my fifth month. In order to get through this period, I had to break down and take a medication for nausea. It was very necessary in my twelfth week, when I needed the strength to read a poem at my friend's wedding. Without the medication I was immobilized. I even had to take a couple of weeks off work by this point because I was so sick. One good thing from this "constant hangover" was that I didn't have to wonder if I was pregnant. Morning sickness, all day long, is a sure sign of a normal pregnancy, right? According to my doctor it didn't guarantee that I would not miscarry, but I preferred to believe that all was well inside of me. By the time I reached my fifth month, I could only feel better by constantly eating throughout the day. I continued to overeat for the next few years. Eating gave me a false sense of comfort and control. As you can see, I didn't live out the new confident ways that I learned in the personal growth program and that really frustrated me because I knew better. I was not demonstrating a significant change in my behaviour.

To help calm my fears about labour and delivery, Ward and I decided to seek some additional help. We hired ourselves someone who had extensive knowledge about pregnancy and delivering of babies. Joanna was a young and gifted Doula, a non-medical assistant who provides various forms of non-medical support in the childbirth process.[1] She was able to answer all of our questions about what to expect even role playing contractions! She was with us for most of the twenty-three and a half hours that I was in labour and delivery. Her main role was to guide Ward about ways of comforting me. After five hours of excruciating contractions, the thought of delivering a mass of seven to ten pounds out of my privates terrified me. I said, "I'm sorry to disappoint anyone but I think I need an epidural." Thank goodness I was past three centimeters, as most moms learn that's how open your cervix has to be in order to receive an epidural! I'm so happy to tell you that I am left with a very positive memory!

WOW! How absolutely remarkable it was to finally meet our "Ella Bella!" And that's what I sang out when she arrived. Very early into my pregnancy I felt that we were having a girl! She came into our lives March 13th, 2006 at 3:30 in the morning. We wondered what she would look like for so many months and here she was at last, a head full of gorgeous hair and that skinny heel that I could feel on the outside of my belly while pregnant!

After the doctors removed the meconium from her nose and mouth before it went into her lungs, Ella was crying for what seemed like hours. Meconium is the first fecal excretion of a newborn child.[2] I remember lying in the labour and delivery room just after putting her to my breast thinking, "Is she going to stop crying?! It wasn't working, she wouldn't breastfeed. Is there anything I can do to help her??" Those were my first thoughts and I still ask those questions, just not with as much worry!

As remarkable as the feeling was to deliver a healthy baby girl, it wasn't long before I started to feel, again, a looming sense of failure. I was not able to comfort my own daughter very well at all, and for many months to follow. I knew what I needed to do. I had the right tools to deal with difficult situations, but I just didn't have the energy to follow through. My emotional health took a dive until I was in the deepest rut of my life. I was running on primal emotions to live each day, mostly fear and anger. The first two years of being a mother was one of the most intense experiences that I have ever been through. The stretching of my comfort zone brought me to a place where I had to face my fears and deal with them, head-on, if I wanted to be a great mom for Ella. I was about to experience one of my most eye-opening adventures in the search for who I was and am, and ultimately, my true-life purpose.

I started a blog, a personal journal on the Internet, in my fourth month of pregnancy because I wanted to share my excitement with my friends and family. I also intended this information to be recorded as a gift for our little Ella Anna. I forced myself to continue writing in the blog even after she was born so that her life was celebrated. It was a way to allow myself to experience motherhood in a softer light. In reality, I was feeling highly insecure, intense anxiety, paranoia, anger, embarrassment and many other ugly feelings. I was paralyzed with fear many times. So, on came the mask! I didn't want everyone to read exactly how I was doing. I didn't want people to perceive me as a bad mother. I didn't want to worry my family and friends. I simply did not want to portray myself as the "monster" I felt I had become. My way of diffusing the negative energy was writing the blog and realizing the positive that was actually around me.

The following are six blog entries that best illuminate my experience as a first time mother in Ella's first year. I struggled each time I sat down to write because I consciously understood that I was not projecting the whole picture, but this was the only way I could safely share at the time.

Underneath each entry I describe what was truthfully going on in my life. I'm now ready to share my real experiences, because I refuse to sit back and be silent! I am able to be honest and use my voice to show others how they can not only survive, but also thrive! So here it is. Here is my reveal.

```
GUESS WHO'S HERE?!!
Sunday, March 19 2006 ~ 12:03 PM
Oh my goodness!  What A WEEK!!! A lot has happened...
```

ELLA ANNA PATERSON is HERE!!!!!

She was born Monday, March 13th, 2006 at 3:30 a.m. She weighed in at 7 pounds and 10.5 ounces and measured just over 19 inches in length. Labour lasted 23.5 hours---crazy!!

I won't go into details, but would like to say that we were surrounded by 'angels' in the labour and delivery room ... the nurses were phenomenal!

And now ... please allow me to introduce our Ella-Bella! She's so so lovely ... in so so many ways!

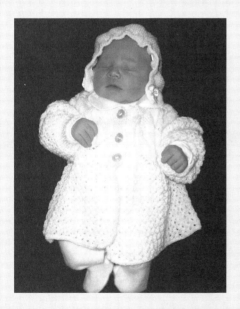

LOOK AT HER!! Ward and I are SO in love! (This is the outfit my Dad bought for us to bring her home in.)

What a week, is right! I was a "train-wreck!" Even though I had an extremely positive experience delivering Ella, which by the way was my worst fear in life, I was terrified to be alone with her. I didn't feel qualified enough to take care of her. I felt like I was thrown into the unknown. This was especially true when a nurse came by with Ella a few hours after delivery singing, "Someone's hungry!" She then left. By this time, I had only slept for one hour in the last twenty-six. "I get so angry when I think about this time, because the nurse offered absolutely no assistance with breastfeeding, and didn't even stay long enough for me to speak up. I didn't even realize that I had a button to call a nurse ... that's how out of it I was!" I read the poster on the wall, and pretended that I knew what I was doing! What I was doing hurt. My nipples were screaming, "This isn't your husband! What's going on here?" Then I finally heard another nurse come into the room and I gathered as much of my polite-voice as possible and asked her to PLEASE show me how to breastfeed my daughter! It turned out that Ella was quite the sucker hence the screaming nipples. One nurse suggested that we use a soother, otherwise Ella would want nursing all the time. My nipples couldn't handle that much use! I also could not find a comfortable feeding position during the entire nine months that we were bonded by breast. The reading I did about raising a child, including breastfeeding, obviously didn't help my situation.

Sleeping was futile during the four days that I was in the hospital. I was that much more weepy and anxious because I hardly slept. Ward was my rock. He was so happy and so proud of our daughter. I never saw him so delighted! I fed on his positive energy as much as I could. When Ward would leave for the night, I felt like a little kid, not wanting him to go. It was quite alarming to me. I was feeling unusually dependent on him. I resorted to being a child, again. How could I take care of my baby in this state?

The fact that I was in the hospital for so long should have been a clue that I was truly having a hard time. The nurses didn't feel that I was ready to go home until I could spend an entire day and night with Ella without much assistance. Their concern fueled my dwindling confidence even more. Finally, we were able to leave on the Thursday afternoon, four days after Ella was born. I was very nervous and extremely full of doubt that I could manage on my own. The nurses were also my support system while in the hospital. Apparently, I needed ten people to raise my daughter.

Also, I have to admit I'm still out of sorts and therefore would explain why I have only updated my website today! However, I am recovering well enough from 'thrush' and sleep deprivation. I finally have colour in my face. But, enough about me ... Ella is just the sweetest little baby ... she loves to make eye contact as best she can, sleeps very well, and eats A LOT! Did I mention Ward and I are in love?!! Speaking of Ward ... he's an absolute PRO at being a father. I see him in a totally different light and LOVE IT! How our lives have already changed. And changed for the better ... we're a family now!

My anxiety level was "to-the-moon," and it didn't help when my mom and Ward would say, "Calm down, because Ella will pick up on your feelings," and I'm thinking, "Well then, this child has no hope at all!" I could not relax. It was impossible. The only time I slept was when I passed out through sheer exhaustion late at night, and then Ella would wake up! It was difficult for me to watch Ella react to what I was feeling because she was not as calm and as comfortable as I knew she could be.

As well as my "to-the-moon" anxiety, breastfeeding remained a toe-curling experience. Thank goodness for an insightful Public Health Nurse. She could see the beginnings of thrush, a contagious disease caused by a fungus that occurs most often in infants and children, characterized by small whitish eruptions on the mouth, throat, and tongue, and usually accompanied by fever, colic, and diarrhea, on each of our bodies.[3] She called the medical clinic to make room for us right away, and to make sure we received the right medication as soon as possible. Use the Public Health Nurses to your advantage. I called any time I needed help with breastfeeding or to see if Ella was gaining weight, or to simply make sure I was doing well by Ella, because everything seemed to be going wrong all around me. I started to break down emotionally. I was crying uncontrollably at this point. The Public Health Nurse asked if I had ever suffered from depression, anxiety or nervousness before pregnancy, because if I had, these next few weeks would bring it out even more. Great, I wanted to "bawl my head off" even more after hearing those words. I felt defeated as a good mother already.

The responsibility of raising a child in the panic-stricken state that I was in brought out all my insecurities; (e.g., Am I worthy of being a mother? Can I really do this? I am SO ugly. Will I ever be happy? Will I start wearing spandex, now? Will Ward stay with me? Will Ella resent me when she grows up?). I was also paranoid that Ella would choke to death or die in her sleep. I also had some horrible visions of hurting her or of others hurting her, and that created such rage inside of me. I really worked hard at not letting those visions or thoughts intrude. I would envision myself burning or whisking them into thin air. To this day I'm quite surprised how naturally this came to me. But I also knew that if I wallowed in these visions, I would really hurt myself, emotionally. All these feelings festered inside me for a good eighteen months.

I felt Ella was better off with Ward and our parents because I was very anxious. It seemed to me at the time that they were able to give her what she needed to be happy. Thank goodness my parents came for two weeks after Ward returned to work. Being alone with Ella was too much for me to take. I actually liked it when Ella was with other people throughout my maternity leave, because she was happy with new people. They weren't frustrated or anxious like me. The responsibility of raising a child frightened me and I was ashamed of this reaction. I was also caught in a vicious cycle. On one hand, I was following the advice of my family and trying to get Ella used to different people. On the other hand, my anxiety made me feel insignificant as a mother, so letting others handle her was fine by me.

Ella was sleeping well, I thought, but she slept in spurts and I later learned that I should have put her in a quiet room for naps, instead of the living room where the television and lights were on. But I also wanted her to get used to noise. I found balancing a healthy atmosphere for Ella challenging. I couldn't have her out of my sight in case she spit-up or something else bad happened. I was extremely paranoid for many months to follow. As a result, I slept with her in bed all swaddled up like nobody's business, or on the couch with her on top of me. After a month, though, she slept right beside my bed in a bassinette with her head propped up so that she wouldn't choke. Ward didn't want to co-share our bed with Ella. I had to wean myself from having to be with her constantly throughout the night which I did in stages. It was fulfilling to feel a sense of family but most times I was envious of Ward's natural ease with Ella. I was so far from feeling a sense of ease, but the love I felt for her was like no other. I was extremely grateful that we could have a child together, considering my first pregnancy ended in miscarriage.

P.S. I do want to take this time to thank everyone who have called our place in the last week and apologize for not returning many of them. I'm hoping this update will suffice for now and just know I will return your calls when I can ... my folks will also be in town for the next two weeks!

Please check the photogallery for more pics!
With much love and thanks to all who have had us in their thoughts,

Elita, Ward, Macykins our Cat & Our Ella-Bella XO

The phone was a huge source of stress for me. I could not multi-task. That meant I had to hold the phone, listen, and then think of a response to say, and then say my response into the phone, all the while trying to keep Ella calm. Difficulty with the phone was such a surprise to me because talking on the phone was always a source of comfort for me. So yes, I was out of sorts. My folks and Ward were my Angels on earth. It was wonderful having my parents visit. I was proud that I finally gave them a grandchild. I just wished I wasn't so cranky and upset around them. Mom and Dad lived in British Columbia many miles away, so we did not see them that often. I felt guilty when I acted this way during our short visits. They kept encouraging me to sleep when Ella was sleeping, but I didn't want to miss out on their visit either. There were times, though, when I'd give in and lie down when Ella was sleeping, but then I couldn't sleep. I could only rest my sore body from breastfeeding and the epidural.

I had no patience! Okay, very little patience. I was abrupt and raised my voice with my parents and Ward if I was rushed or asked to do more than one thing at a time. I was an overprotective "Mama Bear" who couldn't control her snappy responses especially to "Papa Bear," because he was whom I felt most comfortable with, besides my folks. Basically, I was a "bitch-on-wheels," as the saying goes, and hated every moment of it. This behaviour lasted for nearly two years. What I used to effortlessly rely on for relaxation, I couldn't take while breastfeeding, for example: copious amounts of alcohol (not really, just the occasional bottle of wine), chocolate day and night, and melatonin to help me sleep. Let's just say I wish "I" had a soother!

A "MATURE" POOCH LEARNING NEW TRICKS!
Saturday, April 29, 2006 ~ 10:04 am

Well Hellooo!

I have to admit that my updates will be few and far between now that I have the little Ella Bella, but I will try to update as best I can so that Our Bella has stories to read when she gets older.

By this time, Ella was crying nearly every time she ate and for a good three hours in the evening; her witching hours. We were not prepared for such screaming. We even tried all the five "S"s of Dr. Harvey Karp's process with not nearly enough success in our minds! They were, "Shooshing, Swaddling, Side/ Stomach lying, Swaying, and finally Sucking" by using a soother or finger. [4] Very little felt easy or natural when I cared for Ella. I had a difficult time soothing her and I felt nothing was more important than being able to comfort my child as her mother. This experience was crippling for my sense of well-being.

I also had a chronic cough for six years which added fuel to my psychological meltdown. I had coughing spells nearly every twenty minutes. It became even more disruptive because every time I breastfed I would cough until I gagged. On top of all this, the hormones that were released from breastfeeding relaxed my bowels, making me run to the bathroom at the same time. I would have to listen to Ella cry every time I put her down so that I could go to the bathroom. I became very quick in there. I also had to run to the bathroom when we went for walks or the store or while traveling. My bowels were irritated! I could only leave the house when my bowels were good and ready; otherwise, I had an embarrassing accident.

> It really is amazing how much she has already changed in nearly seven weeks of her gorgeous, magnificent life. I fall in love with her more each and every day ... it's amazing watching a miracle grow right in your very arms! She's even starting to look like a little person now! Her hair has grown more ... her cowlick stands so tall and proud!
>
> In the beginning, she ate and ate and ate for hours on end and how my nipples HURT LIKE HECK!!! WOW!!! Then the most caring Health Nurse, Deb, realized that both her and I had Thrush - yeast on my nipple and in her mouth and bum. Well we nipped that situation very quickly and were both better in less than a week ... I've been able to breastfeed her since! (She had to see her doctor four

times in two weeks, the poor thing!) Then her Baba and Deda were down to visit and help for two weeks and what a time we all had! Then shortly after, Grandma and Grandpa Paterson came back from a trip of a lifetime to Peru and Ecuador and had many stories and gifts to share! Ella has also had the pleasure of meeting many friends and family and little people ... a huge thanks to all who took the time to visit!

It was great to have many people around. Being with people made me happier as I saw how much joy Ella brought to them. I was very proud of her but somehow I felt I wasn't showing it. I was feeling so insecure. It came so naturally to others why not for me? I was more comfortable with my friends because I could relate better to them. They were familiar to me. To show them how grateful I was for their support and friendship, I especially tried to be happy around them. This behaviour may have made them think that all was well, when indeed it wasn't. I was just relieved to be in a situation that felt familiar.

Lately she's really enjoying her swing and bouncy chair. She also likes to lie on the couch and kick her legs and arms right out. Ella's going to really enjoy a jolly jumper or something that'll let her use her legs. And how she LUVS to smile!!! I just wish our camera didn't have such a delay. I have yet to capture her smiling away. But I have made a little movie! I'll see if I can upload it on our photogallery. She's been sleeping on average five hours a night and napping in the mornings. Sooo ... I'm not all that sleep deprived, unless I eat salsa or something stupid like that! And how I just LUV kissing her face ALL OVER! Her chubby cheeks are extremely desirable. Speaking of chubby, she's gained two pounds in three weeks and is now weighing in at 10 pounds and 7.5 ounces! She sure is thriving and how grateful we are for that. She's really interested when I sing sentences to her! I don't know any nursery rhymes ... so I better get that into action, eh?! After

typing this last sentence I went onto the internet and found a
really great website http://www.niehs.nih.gov/kids/lyrics and sang
her to sleep. I now have no excuses. She also really REALLY enjoys
it when Ward plays his guitar for her! But two of our favourite
things with Ella is when she falls asleep in our arms and smiles
while staring into our eyes ... these are the most precious gifts
ever. WE JUST LOVE YOU ELLA ANNA!!

And speaking of change ... I've also changed in so many ways. She
is teaching me even more about myself. I now know how an old dog
must feel when learning new tricks!! I've realized just how I like
to be in control and have my life organized and efficient. Well
that's gone out the window!!! (You should see our livingroom NOW!)
Instead, I'm learning to listen to Ella, be patient and trust that
all will be well AND practice, practice, practice! I'm learning
that I have to just DO things with Ella and know that I will only
get better with her! And if we're late...well darn it we're late!!!
(I don't know why it felt okay when it was just me that was late.
Anyway, considering nothing could have prepared me for motherhood
... we're all doing okay! There's even some days I have supper
ready ... I think it's been twice!

My personality was radically changing for the worse. I found motherhood more
difficult than I expected. Before I became a mom I was such a "social butterfly."
I was usually "happy-go-lucky," upbeat and positive. I have come to realize that
these traits were also a mask throughout my life! Very few people witnessed my
true self and the depressive state I was in since a young girl.

When the situation with Ella was out of control the adrenaline would rush
frantically throughout my body. I would sweat profusely, swearing was my new
language, and I had to run to the bathroom urgently! I was afraid to leave the
house. I could hardly comfort Ella at home, what would I be like in public? I
learned to fear Ella's smiling. It meant she was suffering from gas and was about
to have another fit of screaming and crying. We tried traditional medicines

such as gripe water with little success. Even though I was stressed at home, it was still my sanctuary. To this day, there are times when I still get a rush of adrenaline when Ella wakes up crying at night.

I did force myself to get out of the house though and faced the fears by myself or with the few friends I was comfortable with throughout my entire maternity leave. There were times when I was just downright miserable. Sunglasses hid my self-loathing. I was so thankful to my next door neighbour for that suggestion, to wear sunglasses, because it got me out of the house. Her reason though was so she didn't have to put on make-up! I was grateful to her because she had such a down-to-earth attitude, listened so well and used the experiences in her life to try with all her might to understand what I was going through. I also accomplished my goal of getting out of the house by simply walking one house over. We formed quite a lovely relationship, as a result, along with all her other friends I met through the "Splurge Group" I joined during this time. It was a chance for ten women to get together each month to have fun and share money to splurge on themselves! Getting out, for even those two hours, even as miserable as I was, was therapeutic. I continue to "splurge" every month!

Once I got over my reluctance to talk on the phone, it actually became my friend. Now I could talk with friends who had the patience to listen to me complain. It was a huge saving grace for me to talk with my mom over the phone too. There was much distance between us, but at least we could share our thoughts and our love for Ella and each other.

Oh yes, before I part ... I do want to mention our parents, again ... both sets have been absolutely amazing with their support and love for Ella. Ella will never be without. Until my next update ... I hope everyone is doing well and enjoying the springy weather!

With love and new tricks up her sleeves, Elita

p.s. If I haven't said it enough...our Wardnick is an exceptional father. He's patient, a good listener, and remains to be a calming energy in both our lives. He also loves bathing and changing her and just BEING with her. I can leave the house and not worry one bit, because I know Ella is with her father who loves her more than he's ever loved and isn't scared to do anything with her! I'm learning a lot from just watching him.

p.p.s. If any of you new moms find your child gassy...contact a chiropractor who specializes in infants. We went to Dr. Nelson on 13th and had him work on her body, as birth is extremely stressful on their wee little bodies! After Dr. Nelson gently worked on her back – she had one vertebra out – she was so much happier! Until I eat the wrong foods! And speaking of birth being hard on babies bodies ... it's also a good idea for the chiropractor to look at your post-partum body. I'm already experiencing pain-free hips,

We realized that reaching out for various kinds of medical help would make a difference with Ella's crying, so we took her to see a chiropractor. His treatment and suggested burping technique helped, somewhat, but a week after taking Ella to see him, she started crying all over again. The chiropractor was so much calmer than us. Ella responded well to him. In my follow-up appointments he would ask me how Ella was doing. I lied about her behaviour because I was ashamed of my inability to have the same calming effect on Ella as he did.

"SLEEP BEGETS SLEEP"
Monday, May 29, 2006 ~ 11:05 am

*****
Yes ... not sure if I mentioned before that our Little Ella Bella was still crying in the evenings up to several hours a night?! But she was. Even with going to the chiropractor - but at least she wasn't crying every time she was finished eating with gas

pains. Anyway, I was sharing my woes with my dear friend, Carla, and she mentioned to me a book by Kim West called "Good Night, Sleep Tight". She said the techniques mentioned in the book made her daughter a very HAPPY baby! Weeeellll ... I bought that book as quickly as I could and started Ella on a flexible sleeping schedule! I didn't realize just how important it was to create a bit of structure for my pum'kin! So now...I just watch for signs of sleepiness (yawning, rubbing of eyes, unexplained crying, etc.) and put her down when she's still drowsy so she can fall asleep on her own, and sometimes watch her fall right to sleep or I stand by to let her know that I'm there for her when she cries out. Otherwise, she's now averaging eight to ten hours of sleep a night and napping four times a day!

I'd like to let you all know that our daughter is now one of the happier kids on the block!!

Ella still had bouts crying! I was even more miserable and angry at this time because we would try different techniques to calm Ella, but nothing seemed to comfort her. It was becoming unbearable. I started to have fits of rage. I became another person. I would clench my teeth, my hands would form fists, my face would turn red, my body would start to vibrate and the whole time I would be hysterically shrieking through gritted teeth. I basically had an adult temper tantrum. Pinching Ella's diaper or squishing her arm tighter than normal would bring me back to reality. Sometimes, I'd shove her down on the couch or crib or bed and either have a fit with her in the room or just leave her there. Then there were others times that I just wanted to shake her so that she would have a "real" reason to cry. "Why are you crying? I fed you! I changed you! We played! You rested! Why won't you stop crying?" I tried everything that I had read and heard but it wasn't working!

I understood how people could shake their babies. The pressure and stress in these situations is unfathomable. How frightening it made me feel to think I was so close to that. I was so close to hurting, or even killing her. Somehow I found the strength to not go that far. I knew I could not live with myself if I did anything to hurt Ella like that. This whole experience has helped both Ward and I have a stronger appreciation for single parents. I cannot imagine how difficult it must be to go through such anxiety and frustration alone.

I was left with incredible shame and guilt for days after these episodes of rage. I would pray to my Guardian Angels to please help me with the emotional breakdowns that scared the "living daylights" out of me. I felt controlled by them. I still ask for help from my Angels today. I would also ask myself, "How am I supposed to teach my daughter to manage her emotions, when I am out of control?" What was even more alarming was that yelling at Ella felt like the most natural thing in the world. My mom was a "loud speaker" and would get quite frustrated with my brother and I when we were kids. I didn't like being yelled at back then, and I was extremely worried that I would cause the same anxiety in my daughter. I just hoped that this behaviour would eventually pass. It didn't. I became an extension of my mom. Raging became a way of life for another year. Now that I am a parent, I understand where my mom came from and why she did what she did. She was young, she was scared, and she was frustrated. She did her best considering her life circumstances. I am thankful my parents did their best with what they knew. We now nurture a healthier and honest relationship – a friendship. This is a gift that means the world to me, and Ella will benefit too.

I wouldn't talk very much with Ella because I wanted to stop the negativity from spewing out of my mouth. I was resentful because my experience was nowhere near my romantic notions of motherhood. Really the most romantic notion I had was to hold and comfort my baby. I didn't think this was asking for too much. I constantly felt that I should be a better mom and I wasn't rising to the occasion.

Ward and I were constantly on each other's nerves due to lack of sleep, not dealing well with Ella's blood curdling screams, and my on-going anxiety attacks. We would tell each other to calm down so that Ella wouldn't pick up on our stress. I hated my tone of voice with Ward. It was short and snappy and just downright disrespectful. It also didn't help when I forgot nearly every third word I wanted to say. If he didn't hear me the first time and I had to repeat myself, I would be rude, and talk "slooowly and LOUDLY." Ward got the brunt of all my stress. My fits of rage did not escape him, either. I felt that he just didn't understand what I was going through and that was the most frustrating part of all. I just wished he could read my mind, but he couldn't read it before, so what made me think he could now? I understood "madness" at this point in my life. The sensible part of me was void of comfort and commonsense.

Describing this behaviour in such detail is painful and leaves me feeling extremely vulnerable. However, I strongly believe that someone out there is going through the very same thing and I want her to know that she is not alone! There is help surrounding you. Your illness can heal with patience, the will to change and professional guidance.

```
JUNE UPDATE : )
Friday, July 7, 2006 ~ 9:07 pm


*****

Just a wee update...June was a marvelous month!! Ella became three
months and started to become that much calmer and happier! She
got back into her sleeping rhythm, but still wakes up later in
the evening to fall back to sleep around 11:00 pm if not later.
Oh well...she's like her mama who's a night owl. Ella is also now
using an exersaucer and a bumbo now that she can hold her head up
straight and tall - thanks to Auntie Gerri and Jan! She is also a
slobber-machine ... and a puker! Thank goodness for the eleventeen
bibs we received as gifts! Then there's her singing and smiling
when she gets up. She sleeps so well through the night and even
```

```
takes a couple naps in the morning at two to three hour stints!
That's my girl!! Anyway, she's healthy, continues to giggle like
an old man and is all about the bib! We're sooo proud of you Ella
and love you SILLY!!
Hope everyone is enjoying the blue skies and puffs of cloud
 ~ XO


p.s. Check out <http://www.flickr.com/photos/littlewardorelita>!
```

I was feeling better at this time because the extra sleep made a difference in Ella's and my behaviour. My outlook was more positive. Ella and I were able to take walks outside and enjoy the fresh air. Taking a trip to visit my folks and visiting more with other family and friends helped me overcome some of my fears about parenting. Ella was much more resilient than I thought, and so was I. I learned that I could, in fact, nurture my "Bella" even a little bit. We even moved her to her own room and crib when we all returned home! This was a huge step for me. I was starting to trust myself a little more and trusting that Ella would be okay. I had to have the mask on during these visits, so that I could get through them. I felt that as a new mother it was my duty to share and showcase my new bundle in my hometown. I believed that we had to appear as if we were the ideal family. No one could have imagined what we were going through at the time.

Once I returned home, my friends worried more and more about my condition. I started to decline their invitations to go out with them because Ella's naptime was a priority. My friends strongly encouraged me to join them at one of the mom's meetings at the YMCA, in an effort to get me out of the house. However, I could tell right away that I didn't belong there. Everyone was sharing stories of how well their babies were sleeping and crawling and doing math, and then I shared how grateful I was for even getting out of the house and showing up! The rest of the time, I was praying that Ella wouldn't start crying in front of everyone. It was very intimidating to be around mothers I perceived as perfect. This comparing extended to other mothers as well.

Ella's crying continued to be a huge source of anxiety for me. I would make sure I was right there to stop her from getting over-stimulated every time that she was about to cry. This usually meant putting her soother back in her mouth. This behaviour would catch up with me down the road. The first three months of Ella's crying truly affected my emotional health. I felt this must be similar to what soldier's experience when they return home sick with post-traumatic stress disorder. The adrenalin rush I would feel as soon as I heard her fuss would spiral my anxiety to a higher level.

Thankfully, my friend Carla, with whom I worked with briefly and then became friends with, was there to help me through these tough times. She shared her wealth of knowledge and experience that she had gained from raising her own daughter. Carla became a large source of validation and calm for me because she could relate better to my behaviour and my issues with Ella. She was good at challenging me when I was having a self-pity party and I learned they weren't helping me one bit. She was my reality check. She was able to stop me when I was acting like a victim. Hearing similar words from Ward made me defensive and I reacted negatively. These self-pity parties came, especially when comparing myself to other moms, including my own and Ward's, and when I compared Ella to other babies. Now as I reflect on this, it was one of the worst things I could have ever done. I was not honouring who we were.

In order to cope with motherhood and be present with Ella, it was common for me to ask myself, "How would I feel if Ella were to die?" This would shake me to the core and bring me back to gratefulness for my family. I felt remorse every time I asked that question, but at the same time I felt relief knowing that I felt tremendous pain at the thought of losing Ella. These feelings helped me recognize the bond between us. I was reassured that all the anxiety and stress that I was going through was all worth it.

DATES TO REMEMBER!
Thursday, November 30, 2006 ~ 1:11 pm

*****

Wednesday, November 8th – Ferberizing/no more Soothers
Well ... by now you've all read how we were trying to do 'the shuffle' with Ella because she was still waking through the night. Well, her night-wakings were getting worse as the month progressed. She'd get up twice a night for at least 1 to 2 hours screaming/crying, it was awful, awful, awfulness. Sooo...through sheer desperation, Ward called his Mom at the YMCA and she got a book from Sally Elliott by Dr. Richard Ferber and read it to us for an hour as we sat in the livingroom. Everything that Marion read was EVERYTHING we were going through. And the one sentence that made me see the light was, "When putting your child to sleep, ensure the environment is the same as when baby would wake in the night." Now, I know Kim West wrote the same advice, but when you're sleep deprived for nearly two months, a person changes and your brain doesn't work quite the same way, and it's not nice. Just ask poor Ward and my counsellor. Anyway, we started "ferberizing" Ella that night because we knew something HAD to work for her. It was also the last day she would have her soother as it was waking her up at night and not providing any comfort whatsoever. More importantly, we finally released ourselves of the "sleep crutch". Let me tell you, however...you have to be ready to hear your baby scream. You need support. Ward was WONDERFUL; he held my hand and kept telling me over and over that everything was going to be okay. At one point, Ella cried for 2.5 hours before finally falling asleep at 5:30 a.m. to sleep-in till 7:45 a.m. (Know that we did check in on Ella at interval times!) The next night ... not a PEEP! The following nights were just as positive. And if she did wake up, she put herself to sleep. If any parents out there want more info, call! I do have to say that Kim West's "shuffle" did prepare us for this step!

Marion ... thank you SO much for reading to the both of us that night ... you were tremendously sweet to do that. Did I tell you that I find it VERY relaxing when people read to me.

I was finally opening up a lot more to the world. I started to lift my mask. I couldn't keep writing as though I was wearing "rose-coloured glasses!" People needed to know more of what was really going on. This was our life. I needed to be real. I tried as best as I could to be honest and comfortable with what I wrote. I'm relieved that I found the confidence to write, because it felt invigorating to share more of the truth. Being creative was my outlet for pain. Working on the blog and photo gallery were some of the more energizing and healing things I could do for myself.

By this point, I had struggled alone for over six months. I was of the mindset that if I "thought" myself to this point in my life, I could surely "think" my way out of it. My negative thinking combined with my apparent lack of coping skills caused me to assume that I was simply a poor mother? Who wants to admit to that? I sure didn't. I desperately wanted and needed someone to tell me, "Elita, you are just struggling right now. It's all going to be okay. You don't need to do this alone. I know what to do to help you."

I hit rock bottom and became this woman who felt numb to anything that used to make her laugh and feel good inside. A woman who had became a shell of the person that she used to be. I could not take the sleepless screaming nights and Ella's nearly nap-less days, anymore. Rock bottom came soon after I returned from spending a month in British Columbia with my folks. Ella woke up two to three times every night while there to breastfeed for ten minutes and then cry for twenty. I was extremely sleep deprived. I was miserable even being around my parents, people with whom I was most grateful to have in my life. Flying home alone with Ella screaming, in my already shriveled state, intensified my Postpartum Depression and was another factor that led to my hitting rock bottom.

Ella was now seven months old. We began the battle to train her to sleep through the night. Each week got worse for our family because the training wasn't working and Ella could not be calmed. I spent most of my time watching television to escape. I ate large amounts of food saturated with sugar and fat because it gave me instant relief. I was becoming a recluse and spoke with very few people, mostly Ward or my mom. Ward did what he could to help and still get enough sleep to work each day. He would come home at lunch to take Ella and give me a break. I couldn't stand being out of control anymore. My mom started to call more than once a day to check up on me. She even called Ward at work and asked if she should visit. I finally surrendered! I accepted my mom's support. I was finally ready to admit that I was struggling, and that it was not a weakness to accept help. I needed to tell the truth!

I started down the road to recovery. My mom came to support me for the next three weeks. Ward insisted that I see a professional counsellor, which I did. I also went to see my doctor about taking an anti-depressant, especially after I read the following signs and symptoms of Postpartum Depression on the www.BabyCentre.com website. These were insomnia, weepiness or sadness, diminished interest in once pleasurable activities, difficulty concentrating, change in appetite, anxiety, moodiness and irritability, withdrawal from family and friends, excessive guilt, panic attacks, and finally suicidal, scary, or constant negative thoughts.[5]

I fought asking for medications until now because I found that, in the past, the side effects from prescription medications were often as bad as the symptoms I had been suffering. However, this time I was terrified about progressing to suicidal thoughts, which were inevitable if I continued the way I was going. My doctor informed me of the side effects, the length of time I would have to be on the medication and the cost. She then tested my hormonal levels because for some people Postpartum Depression may be directly affected by a hormone imbalance. My hormone levels were normal. I was shocked! I really was crazy all on my own. We giggled a bit, even though I found the results frustrating. She was pleased that I was already seeing a counsellor and that my mom was visiting. That's how my consult ended. My true medical condition went undiagnosed and no other recommendations were made. In retrospect, I realize that I could have used my voice to insist on more information, help and support from specialists and health care providers, including support groups.

I found out later that unbalanced hormones are not the only contributing factors to Postpartum Depression. I learned as well that genetics or heredity plays a huge part, along with your environment, as does your overall perception of yourself. I was a great candidate to develop Postpartum Depression but I really had no reason to believe that I was suffering from the illness because of the hormone results I had received.

Tania, a good friend who was coping with her own struggle from a severe form of Postpartum Depression, was constantly asking me to join her at the regular Postpartum Depression Support group meetings at the YMCA. Obviously, she recognized something that I didn't. My thoughts were, "I didn't have a psychotic episode. I wasn't on any medication. I wasn't even diagnosed with having PPD; I would be making a mockery out of all of you!" It worried me that the one person who truly could relate to my condition was Tania. No one else in my life really understood what I was going through but her.

I can't tell you how much quicker I would have healed if I had attended those meetings, instead of just the counsellor that I was seeing at the time. I could have used a group setting with other moms who were struggling and learning coping strategies together. I was stubborn about looking after my own needs. Ella's sleep problems were way more important to me. If she didn't get her sleep during the day, we all paid for it at night with even more screaming. We learned a year later that she was having night terrors, a sudden awakening associated with a sensation of terror, occurring in children, especially those of unstable nervous constitution.[6] I discovered that lack of sleep is the main contributor to night terrors. Having a routine was essential for both Ella and I.

Ward and I were desperate to find solutions for our parenthood dilemma. Ward's mom found a very useful book. Richard Ferber's "Solve Your Child's Sleep Problems," really resonated with us. He talked of what parents went through with children who didn't sleep well. We were feeling exactly what he wrote; "The parents are tired, frustrated, and often angry. Their own relationship has become tense, and they are wondering whether there is something inherently wrong with their child, and whether they are unfit parents. In most cases the parents have had lots of advice from friends, relatives, and even their pediatrician on how to handle the situation. 'Let him cry; you're just spoiling him,' they are told, or 'That's just a phase; wait until she outgrows it.' They don't want to wait, but they are beginning to wonder if they will have to, since despite all their efforts and strategies, the sleep problem persists. Often the more the parents try and solve the problem, the worse it gets. Let me assure you there is help." [7]

We felt so much hope! Ward was feeling so encouraged that he finally opened up and told me about his own depressive feelings that had been brewing inside of him for some time. I was astonished to hear that he was having as hard of a time as I was. But why wouldn't he? Ward was dealing with a wife who couldn't control her emotions anymore. He had to stay strong for both Ella and I. I felt so badly for him and gave him a huge hug – a real sincere and loving hug. Allowing each other to be this vulnerable deepened the connection between us.

Saturday, November 11 - Drinking from the bottle again, "WOW!" what freedom for Mom, again!!! Otherwise, I was attached to Ella every three hours and was lucky if she ate for a minute … ARGH!

YES!!! What a sight it was to see Ella drinking from her bottle again!!! Not only was her darn soother stopping her from sleeping, it was stopping her from enjoying her bottle, again. Now, I certainly am not a parent against soothers. And I didn't care if Ella had one until she was eleven, but boy am I glad that we finally found the reason why she didn't want it for a couple months. What freedom I feel!!

There were not enough exclamation points to describe my relief when Ella started drinking from the bottle, again. She was only breastfeeding for a couple minutes at a time for nearly two months. She was miserable as a consequence and, yes, I was worried. I know, "big surprise." I assumed the soother was a "crutch," but I never thought it would stop her from wanting the bottle! This was a scary situation because Ella was losing weight and became too distressed to sleep. In retrospect, the stress was likely causing a lack of milk production, and Ella's appetite was not being met.

Saturday, November 11 – Husband & Father of the Year

I am one of the most fortunate women on earth. Seriously. On Ward's own accord, he booked me a suite at the Delta Inn on the above noted date. He not only booked me a suite with down-everything, he also booked me a room on a floor that did not allow children!

WHAT
A
MAN!!!

Theeen I was able to get a magnificent massage by my very talented massage therapist and dear friend, Karry Sali; eat all the junkfood on earth, and then watch a girlie movie to then have the crappiest sleep ever. Oh well, sleeping till 9:30 a.m. to a delivered breakfast made up for it all!! And even though I felt slightly nauseous leaving my hubby and babe that night, I thoroughly recommend that every Mom receive this treatment … at least ONCE A MONTH!

Ward, I thank you from the bottom of my stressed-out heart for such an experience. I still have such great memories of the room and breakfast! XO

Ward booked me a hotel room at the Delta Inn for some much needed "me" time, and I was beyond elation. I was overly giddy and made myself nauseous.

I suspect though, that Ward probably just wanted an evening to himself and his daughter. Ella was usually happier with daddy. He was calmer than mommy, that's for sure. I was amazed how much I enjoyed myself and wished I had another night.

Sunday, November 12th – Ella's first cold that lasted over a week

Yup … I survived Ella's first illness without a bump! She had a very runny nose and coughed a bit at night and survived well, all thanks to Jan for recommending Dimetapp. It was also funny how Ella would make her tongue cup under her nose so she could catch her nose-drool. She sooo HATED us cleaning her nose with Kleenex. She just hates her face being cleaned all together. But we just clean it anyway, we can't have a baby of ours eating nose-drool for breakfast, lunch and dinner and have nose-drool-on-lookers everywhere.

I was afraid of Ella getting sick because I wasn't sure how I would react. It seemed that I had much to learn about caring for her. When Ella did become sick, I found that I could actually soothe her! This validated that I could indeed comfort her. I found this experience to be very fulfilling. We bonded even more! I finally felt like a mom I envisioned.

Thursday, November 16th – stopped breastfeeding. Mom finally went on a diet full of zest and garlic and wine (!) and already lost 8.5 pounds!!! Check-out http://www.sonomadiet.com

With Ella hardly eating at my breast and losing weight and becoming dehydrated, I finally started Ella exclusively on formula. Not only do I feel freer, I feel saner. I guess having the chance to sleep-in for the last two weeks helps, too ;o) Stopping breastfeeding was a hard decision, but when your daughter is weaning herself and needs more nutrition, it made my decision that much more easier.

I felt the closest to "normal" for the first time in eight months. I wasn't prevented from doing so many of the things that I used to enjoy! Dieting wasn't one of those enjoyments, but I was imposing this experience on myself, intentionally. Ella was now totally weaned. I had one less thing to concern myself about before returning to work.

Friday, November 17th - My Mom came for a three-week stay!! Sleeping-in is the best medicine ever! Laughing is pretty good, too!!

HOORAY! I finally said "YES" to my Mom's request to come out and help with Ella!!! Next best thing I ever did besides "ferberizing" Ella. However, with stopping breastfeeding, having "Aunt Flo" visit for the second time in over a year, and starting a diet, my poor Mom also had to deal with an extra high-strung daughter. But all is much better these days and we're actually enjoying one another's company, again! And just how much Ella loves Baba, too! They are such a match. They play so well together, and Mom adapted quite quickly to Ella's eating and sleeping schedule! Baba also taught Ella how to "cluck" her tongue and clap her hands! And how Ella can shop with Baba and I, she's so happy to watch people go by and look at all the pretty Christmas decorations while riding in the front seat of the cart!

Mom … thank you for being such a wonderful Baba! If only Ella could remember these days when she grows up! Dad …thank you for letting go of Mom for three whole weeks and for the Costco trip!!! You're a pretty wonderful person, too!

My mom arrived! She totally gave of herself and she respected our decisions and choices. My dad sacrificed by being without mom for nearly a month. He was always so helpful researching information that helped us raise Ella. We weren't sure what we would have done without the both of them. During this particular time, my paranoia was severe, and I thought that Ward and my mom were plotting against me. I remember yelling to them downstairs when I was breastfeeding Ella in her room, for them to stop talking about me. They didn't know what to say! How could they understand my yelling when all they were talking about was her trip out and if she wanted flavoured cream in her coffee?

Tuesday, November 28th - second Kindermusik class of 8 weeks … all about animals!

Although, it took Mom, Ella and I 25 minutes to get to class because of the terrible Albert Street road, and could only enjoy the last 20 minutes of the class, Ella had SO MUCH fun!!

Thank you Baba and Deda for helping with the cost!

I also have to mention just how much Ella LUVS her "Baby Signs" DVD. It captivates her for the entire 20 minutes!! She'll learn how to sign for "book", "duck", "dog", "cat", "hat" and "all gone". And just for an experiment, I also tried another DVD from the Baby Einstein collection, and it did not receive the same attention, whatsoever. Interesting!

Thank you Gramma and Grampa Paterson for such a worthwhile gift and always being your generous selves!

Visit http://www.flickr.com/photos/littlewardorelita/ for more pictures!

Singing actually made both Ella and I happier and I felt I was doing something positive with her. Singing got us through diaper changes, bath times, car rides, and low times in the day. I began voice lessons in the Spring of 2007; about a year after Ella was born. This has been a desire of mine since high school, because singing felt so good for me.

> Baba has left the building ... but will be returning in a month!!
>
> ... and we're ALL so very much REVITALIZED for it!!
>
> THANK YOU SO MUCH, BABA, for taking the time to visit with us and help us all feel better! You gave me the time to clean the house, sleep-in, cook for you and Ward ... lots, drink coffee and chat with you in the mornings, enjoy an evening or two with the Warden ... simply put ... you gave me the time to enjoy life, again! Also, Ella has been sleeping so well and is happy as a Pig-in-Poo! She so loved being with you!!

My mom and I enjoyed relaxing mornings with coffee, chatting and watching morning talk shows while Ella was napping. It was like having a pajama party. These are some of my favourite things to do with mom, besides shopping!" One morning was particularly uplifting when we were watching "The Ellen DeGeneres Show" and as her guest, Bob Proctor, started talking about the book, "The Secret."[8] I was on the computer at the time and without a second thought, I bought the book online, and then the movie afterward. Listening to their stories was very compelling because I've believed in what they were talking about for a long time, but could never quite tap into the theory's full potential. Some time later, the other authors of the book were on Oprah. It was so inspirational to watch. I felt these shows and the book were signs that I was on the right track to recovery. They gave me hope. The book's premise on how to attract what you desire was so very appealing to me and was easily explained. I wanted peace and purpose. I'm reaping the results more each day!

I wasn't hiding anything here! These experiences really taught me just how much we are mirrors of one another. Ella immediately noticed and reacted to my emotions. How could she rest at this time when I couldn't? How well could Ward cope with my depressed state when he was constantly "saving" us? Of course, he would have his own emotional upheaval at the same time I did.

When Ward and I agreed and were consistent, Ella always reacted well and still does. When we finally decided to "bite the bullet" and let Ella cry, she benefited the most. She was finally able to soothe herself, by herself with no soothers, no rocking, no music, no "shooshing," no putting her on her back in her crib, etc. We eventually learned to not respond to her crying because we knew she was alright, she was in no harm. She was just angry that we weren't playing with her! Once I had gathered the energy to catch my breath, eat properly, care for myself emotionally and mentally, everyone around me reacted favourably. I even started to give Macy, our cat, more loving attention. Life was looking up.

```
NEW YEAR WITH MANY CHANGES ...
Monday, January 22, 2007 ~ 7:01 PM


Well ... Ella's crawling is cute as ever; she's talking up a storm
while pulling herself up to standing by using chairs; she just
loved having her Deda for a two-week visit; Baba is staying for
three more weeks; I finally found a caregiver for our Pumpkin and
she only lives minutes away and we can't wait to see how Ella plays
with her daughter, Angelina; she loves picking out her books and
poking away at the characters; she's eating more table food, now,
and drinks a lot more formula and milk; she's continuing to sleep
through the night and having her short naps during the day (but
we're not complaining); she's laughing a lot and loves it when we
twirl around with her and tickle her (!); Ella just LUVS being on
our shoulders; she loves Macy, but Macy does not ... we're having a
tough time letting her go though as she was our first baby; and
then there's me going back to work. And it's actually not too bad
... but that's because Ella is at home with her Baba! But starting
next week, Ella is going to Kristen's for a couple half days so
everyone can get a feel for each other. I also wrote Kristen a few
notes on Ella (okay, more of a manual) so that she can get a feel
for Ella, that way, too! At any rate, everything is going so well!
We just LUV our Ella SO MUCH ... she's such a character and we've
all bonded so well ... it really is the best thing in the world.
Actually, the best thing in the world is when Ella snuggles into
me to drink her 'milka' before bedtime ... sigh!
```

Going back to work actually turned out to be a blessing. In a way, it was my version of a Postpartum Depression support group. I was able to make my Director happy, quickly and effortlessly. I was able to make co-workers laugh. Everything had a manual! Work was my getaway because I was competent at it, and in turn, it was relaxing. I had the energy to be happier and more playful with Ella because work was a respite for me. Weekends became very special times for our family.

Going back to work was not without its struggles. Preparing for my return became even more challenging when my care-giving option, that I thought I had secured, fell through. Our ultimate choice was the YMCA daycare because Ward's mom worked there and we heard only rave reviews about it. The waitlist was as long as my hair and I had to continue searching for another viable option. I can't tell you how stressful it was to find someone to essentially take over our daytime roles as parents. Kristen and her daughter came into our lives. I felt so relieved that we had found the next best option for our "Bella!" Now, the next challenge was finding work clothes that fit my new bulging body! Eventually, returning to work was still not enough to calm my anxieties. They still lingered and I still had a "short fuse" and resorted to drinking quite a bit to take the edge off. Ward and I often fought about how to teach Ella. It was apparent we still needed help.

By now my Postpartum Depression must have been pretty obvious. I was frustrated, paranoid, anxious as ever, delirious, stretched way beyond my comfort zone, and yet, very much in love with my little daughter. Now that I look back, I realized that my anger wasn't necessarily always negative. It took anger to force me to get to the core of my beliefs and thought patterns and finally make me ask with conviction, "If you're that unhappy, then who do you want to be and what do you want to do about it? What will it take to be at peace?" Asking these questions led to a huge breakthrough. I had to envision something different and change the negative self-talk in my head. I found that everything that I was thinking and saying for all those years had actually become my life; (e.g., being obese; feeling lost, lacking self-confidence, etc.). I reflected back to how I felt when I was confident. These feelings counteracted my negative ways of thinking. I felt that I had better start thinking and envisioning what I wanted to feel in my life, now, so that I could reap the benefits sooner than later.

Another breakthrough happened during my physical exam in the Spring of 2007, when the doctor read my medical history form. The way I answered many of her questions peaked her curiosity. She asked if I was depressed. I sat there saying, "I thought that I just gotten over the toughest part of my maternity. Honestly, I have felt tired, struggled with weight, felt rudderless, restless and anxious most of my life." She asked that I take a week to consider if I was depressed and get back to her.

I did some research and learned that it was quite possible that I was in a depressed state. I also asked close friends around me if they thought I could be. My friends reaffirmed my suspicions. I asked Ward, and he didn't even hesitate to say, "Yes." Again, I did not want to resort to drugs, but instead I fretted for a few weeks. Finally, I calmed down enough to gather my senses and follow my instincts. I scheduled an appointment with a psychologist that dealt specifically with couples and people with anxiety, depression, stress, self-esteem issues and post trauma. Ward and I were in this together, and needed to find a way to live with one another, peacefully and meaningful. Ward could provide another point of view. It seemed like we had to experience great pain before we took any action. We know better, now!

Our psychologist listened to my concerns and history during the first appointment, as well as Ward's story. He concluded, simply, that during my childhood years I dealt with stressful situations in a "fight or flight" response. I now had to learn to calm my autonomic nervous system. He taught us a deep breathing technique that really reduced the emotional and physical arousal. I was finally taught a technique I could easily do when I was feeling anxious and frustrated! After practicing, my chest wasn't nearly as tight, and therefore it was a lot easier for me to breathe deeply and reason. The breathing technique helped me de-stress so that I didn't vent my anger onto Ella and Ward nearly as much. I did not want to be either verbally or physically abusive to Ella just because I never learned practical coping skills to deal with stress. As a rule, when we all got home from work and daycare, we took fifteen to thirty minutes to breathe and relax, so that we could continue with our evening on a happier note.

The psychologist also stressed how important it was for Ward and I to "team-develop" on our finances and self-care. He taught me to be "assertive" rather than "passive-aggressive" where I would become quiet and expect the other person to know what I was feeling and what I wanted. It was important for to me to be direct and describe my feelings and needs, not only at work but in all my relationships. He understood me in less than one hour! I was given knowledge as to why I reacted to stress the way I have all my life. Ward's physical and emotional presence in the sessions was completely the support I needed. He provided an objective point of view and I didn't have to explain the sessions back at home in broken phrases because I kept forgetting words (a symptom of my stress levels). I was a terrible storyteller. Ward would always ask me to start from the beginning and make sure I gave him a plot. Seeing our psychologist was a profound breakthrough for me and for us!

I was still having problems with coughing even though my stress levels were getting somewhat under control. I was desperately looking for ways to fix this problem. It was driving myself and Ward crazy. In desperation, I finally booked an appointment with a homeopath. I heard about him several different times and I followed my instinct and booked an appointment. Doctors I had approached throughout the years could not help me. In fact, I was told several times that I would most likely cough the rest of my life because it's dry in Saskatchewan! I was most certainly not going to settle for that answer! The homeopath confirmed my inability to cope with stress and that my cough was a result of unhappiness, anger and sadness that was transferred onto me through my mother's eighteen year old womb! Yes ... quite unorthodox and not what I was expecting! He went on to explain that my cough was my body's way of crying and coping the best way it could. My body was not built to cope with stress at all. My inability to cope with stress showed up in many other forms such as constant sighing, being very sensitive to temperature, light, sound, many foods, and people's perceptions of me. These symptoms all told a story about the pain I carried inside. Instead of just prescribing something for my cough, he wanted to deal with the root cause of my issues by prescribing a homeopathic remedy that would calm my body, so it no longer needed to cry for help all the time. After taking the remedy dutifully for two months, a miracle happened before my very eyes. I stopped coughing! Well, I now cough maybe 10% of my life away versus 90%, and the wrenching tightness in my chest is gone! Another positive result from the calming effect is my less cranky bowels! I continue to take this remedy when I am sick or when I'm about to do something that will be stressful.

We started applying our knowledge from our marriage counselling sessions and the homeopathic remedy. Ward and I found a new deeper openness in our relationship. It allowed us to talk more freely about how we truly felt and thought. During one of these discussions, we reached an epiphany together. The truth was I did not allow him to empathize with me because I did not believe he meant what he was saying! My not believing and trusting Ward meant that I was not respecting him and his efforts to help our recovery. I did not believe in, trust or respect myself either. We finally understood the underlying reason for our constant irritation with one another. This was quite an awakening for me. Our relationship was the one I struggled with the most. I now say, "I believe in myself and I trust in you Ward" when we are disagreeing, or I just leave the room! Although our relationship still needs work, the words, "I apologize" or "I'm sorry" are much more regular in our household. Healing happens so much quicker when your body is relaxed.

We decided that Ella could benefit from seeing the homeopath as well, so off we went just after her second birthday. The homeopath's impression of Ella was also an eye-opening experience. I filled out a history form for her, and then he asked more questions about my pregnancy, labour and delivery, and Ella's behaviour when she was a newborn. I went on to explain that I was quite excited and worried during my pregnancy because labour and delivery were my greatest fears in life. When Ella was born we knew that there were complications due to meconium being present when my water broke. This gave the homeopath a clue that Ella had experienced trauma in my womb. I also went on to explain how her head was lodged in my pelvis for almost twelve hours during labour. He said that her little body was remembering all of these events, which in turned explained her night terrors and her inability to be soothed. The trauma also affected her disposition in that she cried a lot and got frustrated easily. Ella sounded a lot like me. He prescribed one drop of a homeopathic remedy in her water everyday to relax her traumatized little body. With this new regime, Ella's nights are no longer riddled with restlessness and bouts of screaming, except when she's sick or teething. We are now able to calm her.

As I build supports in my life, I am doing the same for Ella. I attend Angel Therapy counselling sessions to gain a holistic view of our lives and receive ideas to enhance our experiences. Ward and I have also received more counselling on how to parent and deal with Ella's developmental stages. We share our new knowledge with Ella's caregivers at daycare so that, together, we can help her feel calmer and secure in her surroundings. Each of these supports has enhanced our parenting skills and strengthened our bond with Ella. We have come to accept that Ella is quite a feisty little person. She's simply strong-willed, clever, knows what she likes and doesn't, highly intuitive and needs to have choices in her life. After all, these are attributes that will serve her well as an adult and we want to continue instilling them in her, but in a more harmonious way! Ella is here with her own lessons to learn and so her healing continues as will ours.

I honestly do not feel it is an accident that many women go through postpartum difficulties. Rather, it's a symptom of all the hurt, the pain and the confusion that we have experienced throughout our lives and haven't faced. It's an opportunity for us to heal existing issues, so we can become that healthy and whole person that guides the way for our future generations. I'm not sure where I would be now if I had never gone through the personal growth program after my miscarriage. Even though I didn't have the energy to use many of the tools that I had learned, the training made me even more aware of what my life "could be," which was my saving grace. Otherwise, I suspect my situation would have become much worse and perhaps I could have ended up needing extensive psychiatric treatment. I think postpartum illnesses are just symptoms of a larger problem in this world. Much healing needs to be done by letting go of things we cannot control and enjoying what the Universe/God has gifted us all with – "peace" within ourselves through taking responsibility for our actions. It is commonly felt within our circle of friends that the healing starts with the mother. Ultimately, I feel that all of us, not just mothers, need to heal and transform ourselves so that we can change the world to be a better place, together.

I found that once I began my healing journey, it only took focusing on and healing one issue to open the door to heal another. I inspire to live a life where my issues are no longer overwhelming but rather a simple process of being aware and letting go. I feel the purpose of the healing process is to have more peaceful and calm moments instead of chaos and self-judgment. I feel that we should keep in mind that when we are raising our children to be independent, that we teach them "how to ask" for help and to know that it is healthy to do so. They need to set their pride aside and realize that it is not a weakness to ask for help. It's all about setting our children up to win, even if their lives become traumatic.

I believe that in today's society we tend to let problems build-up until the only option is to react to them. It is my hope that my story will show the necessity to think pro-actively about parenthood. That is, look at each individual's life before bringing a baby into this world. You may want to ask yourself, "Are we having children for the right reasons?" I believe women and men should look at what needs to be resolved in their lives and take the steps to heal before having children. Once pregnancy has happened there are many tools that could be used to help determine problems with depression. I think it is a good idea that nurses screen mothers for PPD when they bring their babies for immunizations, if they don't do so already.

As a result of living a very reactive life, it took me to survive a "Hellish" experience to finally deal with what was the root of my "dis-ease" for so many years. Continuing with my healing journey is the greatest gift I can ever pass onto my "Ella-Bella."

The healing possibilities excite me!

So where am I now?

I am a woman on a journey with more meaning and confidence.

I am a woman with a purpose to live as a role model for her daughter.

I am a woman who is comfortable being genuine with herself and others.

I am a woman who believes in herself and acts on her dreams.

I am a woman who continues to fall deeply in love with her husband.

I am a woman who continues to nurture a healthy relationship with her parents.

I am a woman who is compassionate.

I am a woman who is grateful for all she is and for all she has co-created.

I am a woman who is "learning from joy" instead of pain.

I am a woman transforming herself for the greater good.

I am a work-in-progress!

May we all stand in our power with ease!

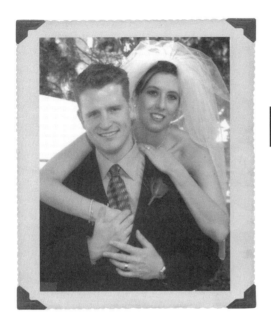

Tania's wedding photo

Tania after giving birth

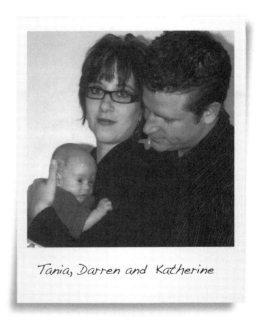

Tania, Darren and Katherine

Chapter Three
Tania's Truth

You cannot change the wind, but you can change your sail.

~ Anonymous

I met my future husband at the ripe old age of twenty-five. We were married in October 2004 after dating for five years. We picked this date so that I would not be thirty when we wed or an "old maid" as elder generations would say. Darren always told himself that he would be thirty or older when he wed. The time was right.

Four months later on February 14, 2005, Valentine's Day, it began innocently enough. My husband, Darren, and I were having lattes at Cornerstone Café while discussing the first year of our marriage and what we wanted to accomplish. We traveled to many beautiful destinations and had wonderful adventures the five years we dated before marrying. After talking about more traveling and the experiences we wanted to have happen next, we began talking about the possibility of a family. Should we? Shouldn't we? Were we ready?

I was not getting any younger. I was already thirty. If we were going to begin having our family, we best start soon. Besides, who knew how long it would take to get pregnant, right? Hopefully I wouldn't get pregnant too quickly because sex would be fun. Hopefully pregnancy happened quickly enough though, so that we didn't begin to think something was wrong. I became pregnant after only a couple of weeks off birth control. What a wonderful gift. It was incredible; a little baby growing inside, multiplying cells, God's creation at its finest. How blessed we felt.

The pregnancy was normal with morning sickness, afternoon sickness, and evening sickness for the first trimester. I gladly ate rice crackers knowing that this nausea would be over eventually. The doctor was a little unhappy with the amount of weight I gained, "Quit eating like it was for two," he would say. My husband made me drink lots and lots of milk. I don't even really like milk, but it is good for the baby so I drank litres of it. Everything was going great.

I was between twenty-four to twenty-five weeks of pregnancy. It was just prior to July 2005. I was having lunch with my girlfriend, Jill, and she was commenting on how great I was looking. My response back was I was doing great but my feet were really swollen. Shoes were hurting. Jill looked at my feet and saw how puffy they were and recommended that I see the Obstetrician just to ensure everything was all right. I phoned the clinic when I returned to work to set an appointment. What luck, there was a cancellation that very afternoon. So I left work early and drove to the doctor's office. The female assistant looked at my feet and said that this was normal. It happens to lots of pregnant women. It is because you are on your feet all day. I can accept that. Then the doctor came in and said he was going to check my blood pressure and weight to ensure everything was good. He said my weight was not bad, but still a problem. Then came the blood pressure result. It was unbelievably high! He checked the blood pressure a second time on the same arm and one more reading on the other arm to be sure. The doctor looked me directly in the eyes and said, "I don't mean to alarm you but my assistant is phoning your husband right now and you need to go to Emergency room right away. Your blood pressure is much too high." Stunned I said, "Okay." I did not know anything about blood pressure and then I started to cry. I was frightened and scared. What should I do? What does this mean? Well, what can anyone do really? I sat in the waiting room and waited for my husband. So, I waited. About fifteen minutes later, which felt like an eternity, Darren walked through the door. The doctor briefed him and told us that we needed to get going because the Specialists were waiting for us at the hospital.

I convinced my husband to allow me to drive my car back to our condo, because after all, I didn't feel that bad. Our condo was only four blocks from the doctor's office. We hopped into one vehicle and off to the hospital we drove. There was no real rush, no real pressure. I mean, I felt fine. There was nothing to worry about. When we arrived at the emergency desk and as I gave my identification to the admitting person, a nurse walked in and said, "We have been expecting you Tania." It was very strange that they would know my name. "Come with me," she said. I put on the hospital nightgown and hopped onto a delivery bed in the Labour and Delivery Ward. My arm was blood pressure cuffed immediately and was told that the equipment would measure my vitals, as well as baby's every fifteen minutes or so. The nurses were friendly. My belly was strapped with a monitor and they listened for my baby's heartbeat and vitals too. The doctor came in and said that they wanted to keep me in overnight for monitoring, just to ensure everything was okay. I agreed, but drat, I didn't have anything packed for staying overnight, no suitcase, no clothing and no makeup. I gave my hubby a detailed list of items that I wanted and he left for home. Darren came back several hours later with a suitcase, which of course, did not contain what I asked for.

Darren stayed with me until around 11pm then he left to go back to the condo. I am thinking that I could go home tomorrow and everything would go back to normal. By normal I meant morning sickness, afternoon sickness, and evening sickness. I phoned work and left my boss a lengthy voice mail message about how I was in the hospital for monitoring. I could not really sleep. The nurses kept coming every hour, or so it seemed. How annoying. There was checking, checking, and more checking.

From then on I was in and out of the hospital. I had two to three days in the hospital and then a couple of days at home. I purchased a home blood-pressure kit. I monitored the blood pressure myself and wrote everything down including the number of kicks I felt from the baby. I really became much more aware of the kicking by then. Work was out of the question and I was given an extended sick leave certificate from the doctor. I kept thinking that this was only a temporary situation. At the very least I believed I would be able to go back to work, box up my stuff and do a decent job of a hand-off to the next person. I was very conscious of this kind of thing. I'm a bit of a perfectionist. I was also beginning a low dose of high blood pressure medication.

My first long-term stay in the hospital took place from July 27th to August 6th. I was twenty-five week's pregnant. I was in a hospital room with three other women. It was very uncomfortable being with three other women whom I'd never met. They seemed nice enough though and we easily exchanged pleasantries. I realized that I might as well get to know them because we were going to be bunked together for quite awhile. It turned out that these women were experiencing complicated pregnancies as well. I thought, "Good. We could commiserate together." The woman right beside me was having problems because the baby was not growing properly. Another woman would be delivering shortly. She already knew and accepted that her baby would be in the Neonatal Intensive Care Unit (NICU). Her first and second babies were also in the NICU. The last woman suffered with gestational diabetes. We had something in common because her husband had Celiac Disease as have I since I was twenty-five years old. I was able to answer the multiple questions she had about diet. It helped take my mind off my hypertension.

During the hospital visit, the obstetrician asked Darren to meet him outside the room to talk privately. I was able to hear the conversation, "My God!" The doctor was having the "your wife or your baby" conversation. He was telling Darren that, "The baby was not really viable this early." Darren was saying. "Save my wife" and in my head, I am screaming, "NO, save the baby!" I've lived thirty beautiful years! I've made many wonderful friends, and memorable life experiences. If there needed to be a choice, I choose the baby. Why wasn't the doctor asking me? Why my husband? Could it be that Darren was more objective or logical? Didn't they recognize and understand the deep connection, the attachment and love I have for this baby that I have been knitting in my womb? Don't I have the power to decide what happens to my body? I have so many hopes and dreams for my baby.

As my blood pressure rose, the medication had to increase. We were in a fight to stabilize my blood pressure. During my hospital stay my blood pressure was as high as 159/106 and it took high dosages of medication over the ten days to stabilize it to 150/90, which isn't even the normal measurement of blood pressure, 120/80.

I was given a needle on August 5th so that the baby's lungs would develop quicker. I was distressed because it was looking more and more likely that I was going to have a pre-mature baby. How could that be? I had done everything the right way. I had taken my folic acid. I drank lots of milk. I took pre-natal vitamins. I even exercised! Life was unfair!

Luckily for me, my mother-in-law, Linda, and my sister-in-law, Sandy, both worked at the hospital. They came everyday to visit during their coffee breaks and lunch hours. I really appreciated their visits. It gave me something to look forward to. They would always ask questions and make me smile and laugh. When I told Sandy who my obstetrician was, she smiled and suggested I change doctors to one who specialized in high-risk pregnancies. She suggested the Obstetrician who delivered her daughter. I was annoyed with that suggestion but didn't say anything to Sandy because I didn't want to offend her. I knew best, right? Wrong!

While my nurse was taking blood pressure one afternoon, my blood pressure rose by five points when I saw my current obstetrician. If that was not an indication to change obstetricians, nothing else was. I looked at the nurse and started to cry, "Please help me. I don't want him to be my Obstetrician anymore," as I pointed toward the hallway where he was standing. Nurses are not supposed to recommend physicians but when I asked, "Hypothetically, if you were having a baby and experiencing problems, whom would you want to see?" Ahah, I got the answer. She recommended a young, knowledgeable, hip female Obstetrician. The nurse told me that she would mention to this Obstetrician that I wanted a second opinion.

It just so happened that this new obstetrician was doing rounds that night. I asked her if she would take me on as her patient. I tearfully told her about the "your baby or your wife" incident. She was clearly empathetic and understanding. She told me she would love to take care of me, but she would be on vacation. She recommended the same obstetrician that Sandy had mentioned earlier, and that he was well respected. She said she learned a great deal from him. Okay, that was now twice that he had been recommended. So I agree. I asked for my chart to be given to my new obstetrician.

I saw my new obstetrician the next day. What a wonderful man and such great bedside manner! He ordered an ultrasound at his clinic which was located in the same hospital. He knew my mother-in-law, Linda, and sister-in-law, Sandy, and agreed to take me as a patient. I think he enjoys a good challenge! I was wheel-chaired to his office that morning. I met his staff who were such nice ladies. I felt welcomed. During the ultrasound, jelly was put on my belly, and then "presto" there was the picture of my baby! My new obstetrician and the ultrasound technician discussed the ultrasound. The obstetrician said that everything looked normal, but he wanted to monitor my urine for protein. He then informed me that he was going to sedate me to get as close to thirty weeks as possible. Great, only five weeks to go! Okay, so now I have a goal to reach and a plan. I was to be sedated to lower my blood pressure. All was good.

I was discharged from the hospital on August 6th, but little did I know that this was only the beginning of a very challenging journey. I was hospitalized again August 11th for one week. In addition to the high blood pressure medications, I was also given Ibuprofen and chewable Aspirin during this stay.

I had ultrasounds almost every day to ensure that the baby was developing appropriately. They would monitor my condition and not intervene unless my condition deteriorated, the baby was compromised or they found protein in my urine. At this time my blood pressure was high and fluctuated (i.e. 140/90 to 120/70 to 150/100), but things appeared to be under control.

Little did I know this was my last hospital stay associated with pregnancy. I was in the hospital from September 3rd to 15th, 2005. Fortunately, I had got a private room this time. The room was quiet and relaxing. It was the farthest room from the nursing station at the very end of the hall. The patient across the hallway, Maria, had pregnancy complications because she had an incompetent cervix, (a cervix that opens pre-maturely under the pressure of the growing uterus and fetus).[1] She was on hospital bed rest for the past six months. I am not exaggerating when I say that she had her legs in the air most of the time. Maria and I became great friends because we were both long-term patients. We were the nurses' pets and they were more gentle and supportive to us than other patients. We were special to them. They encouraged both of us every day and congratulated us every night. All was going well.

Maria and the nurses helped make the days pass more quickly. The nurses knew that I was lonely and they would visit. Maria and I would visit with each other every afternoon for about an hour or so. I would get wheel-chaired to her room and we would eat strawberries or other goodies together. Linda and Sandy visited me regularly. My mom brought her lunch to the hospital and ate with me. My youngest sister, Shirrae, would come and see me when she didn't have university classes. It was all very nice and sometimes, my grandparents would pop in for a visit as well as my aunts and uncles. I really appreciated when anyone would come and see me. My Mary Kay girlfriends, Jill, Tracy and Nancy, even came as well as my Mary Kay customers who are dear friends too. I appreciated it when people came and talked about their lives. It helped me from thinking "woe is me" and feeling sorry for myself. It was refreshing.

Darren occasionally came during lunch hour. He was "the rock" and he came every evening from 5:30 pm onward. When I reflect back on this, I don't really know how Darren did it. He went to work every day, phoned me several times during the day, carried his cell phone with him at all times, was taking a university class and came to see me every evening. This really must have worn him out, but every night he would come in and give me hugs and kisses and tell me how amazing I was for keeping that baby inside. He and I would play cribbage to keep our minds off the baby and the blood pressure. He would crack jokes and keep things light. I would always ask him to snuggle with me in the hospital bed. We are both large people, I am 6 feet tall and round at this point and Darren is 6'4' and 250 pounds. Just imagine the looks we would get from the nurses when they came in to take my temperature and blood pressure, finding the both of us curled up together. Most understood and would just smile.

On September 4th, my Obstetrician recommended that Darren and I be given a NICU tour. It was becoming more apparent that I was going to have an emergency C-section at some point. I remember Darren wheeling me toward the NICU, which is around the bend and up the hall from the Mother and Baby Ward. When we arrived, there were three other couples on the same tour. We were at the end of the group. The waiting room had large glass windows so that you could see inside the unit. I was overcome with emotion because it was way too real for me to deal with. With tears streaming down my face, I looked at Darren and said, "I can't do this." He held my hand and led me back to the wheelchair. I don't remember anything the tour guide said. All I remembered was an awful sinking feeling that I was going to have a pre-mature baby.

At 7:20 pm on September 4th, I was given a medication to encourage the baby's lung development. This was my second and final dose. My blood pressure was erratic and kept creeping upward. On September 5th my blood pressure medication was dramatically increased. The daily ultrasounds were showing that the baby's health was deteriorating. It would be a matter of days before I would deliver. It was inevitable. On September 8th, protein over 1 gram was found in my urine. It was time.

Katherine Evelyn Bird came into this world at 2:59 pm on September 8th, 2005. She weighed 2 pounds, 16 ounces and was delivered by emergency C-section. Katherine was immediately rushed to the NICU doctors and nurses. I've often thought about that day. Darren came to see me late morning. I wondered if he knew I was going to have a C-section that day. Did a nurse phone him? The porter helped me into the wheelchair, and away we went. Darren was wearing shorts, a T-shirt and sunglasses. I was very medicated. Days ran into days at that point. I was taking lots of anti-anxiety medication (Atavin) to keep my blood pressure at bay.

I remember sitting on the edge of the operating table with a pillow and was asked to bend forward. There was a poke in my lower back. The nurses helped me lie down. My Obstetrician was near my feet. There was a sheet draping me from neck down so I could not see anything. I could not see my belly. My feet were in stirrups. Darren was sitting to my right by my head, holding my hand. I was frightened and unaware of what was happening.

I don't remember being cut, but I do remember the Obstetrician reaching in and pulling out Katherine, first one arm, then one leg. She was trying to get away. She knew it was not time. It felt like my heart was being pulled out. Katherine was born. I looked at Darren and said, "I thought we were having a boy." I am asked to name her. I look confusedly at Darren. We did not have a girl's name picked. We were both so sure it was a boy. I mean what else could it possibly be? It was causing me so much distress I thought it had to be a boy. Kenneth Michael was the name. I blurted out "Katherine Evelyn." Where did that come from? They were our grandmother's names.

I felt something horrible happening within my body – a sensation, something negative radiating from my very core. I knew something was not right. I did not feel a sense of relief, in fact, the opposite. Panic was setting into my bones, as if I were close to death. My initial thought was to look at Darren. If I was going to die, his were the last eyes I wanted to see. I did not feel relief. The sensation felt strange or foreign to me. It was an emotion that I have never experienced before. I can't describe it. Something awful was happening. I passed out. In retrospect, my body was alerting me of more serious things to come.

I woke in the recovery room. The nurses asked me if I wanted something for pain. "Hell, yes!" I ached all over from the C-section. I was in a dream, a haze. There was no reality. My mother-in-law and Shirrae were in the recovery room, along with Darren. "What did I want for the pain, Demoral or Morphine?" asked the nurse. I said, "I don't know, I can't think. Just get me something." The nurse was asking Darren how much I weighed and my height, all kinds of crazy medical questions. "Christ, look at the chart!" Darren was really frustrated and began to ask Shirrae if she could answer questions. That was my first realization that my sister was in the room with me. I looked at her and said, "Nice shirt, Shirrae." It was yellow and cheery. I passed out.

When I woke again, I was in a private room in the Mother and Baby Ward. Darren was in the room with me. I was really thirsty. I drank several litres of the water and juice he gave me. Darren helped me sit up by using the bed's remote control. I was in much better spirits. We called our grandparents and our parents. There was a buzz all around. My grandmother, Kay, was very excited that we named Katherine after her. According to my uncle she walked around like a peacock! What an honour to be bestowed. We phoned everyone in the immediate family. Darren left to get a coffee and I napped.

Later that day, my blood pressure rose within dangerous limits, once again. This was discovered after a nurse came to my room to take temperature and blood pressure readings. I was immediately taken to the Intensive Care Unit (ICU). The Intensive Care doctor was being paged. He was a young, attractive, blond-haired man with a pleasant African accent. He wore a red shirt and blue pants. I remember thinking to myself, "He looks like Papa Smurf." He talked to me and apologized because he had to slice open my left wrist and tap into an artery. This procedure is to prevent administering additional needles. It hurt. As it was, I looked like a pincushion from all the endless needles prior. I had an IV going in my right hand. I was given, intravenously, a number of medications to lower my blood pressure.

I had my own nurse, Grace, who stayed at the end of my bed all night. I woke in the middle of the night because my face was itching so bad I wanted to scratch it off. When Grace asked me if I want something for it, all I could do was nod. When I looked at Grace again, she had a halo around her head. I found that comforting and I drifted off again. I dreamt of a man with a beard. He was surrounded in white light. I was sitting at a wooden table across from him. I realized who this was, it was God. I started to cry, pound on the table, and yelled, "I am not ready yet. I can't leave Darren with a baby!" He nodded his head and smiled. I felt comforted and slept like a baby.

All my previous medications were increased. They told me that I was going on a fluid restriction of no more than 1500 milligrams a day. Chest x-rays were ordered. I was given anti-anxiety medication. September 9th, the day after Katherine was born, and I still had not seen her. I was very weak. My lower legs were in a device that puffed up every few minutes so that I wouldn't develop blood clots. I was hooked up to monitors on my chest and had an IV in my right hand. I didn't feel good. I felt like I had been in a battle and lost.

Darren and my parents took turns visiting me. Only two people were allowed in my room at any one time. Darren decided that he was going to stay the night. I looked at him. He looked like he had not slept in a week. He looked like a train wreck. He was wearing a baseball cap which meant he had not showered lately. He had pictures of Katherine but I wasn't interested. I was exhausted. When I woke during the night I felt a sense that death was looming. I woke up Darren. I told him, "Death is nearby. We need to pray for the lady in the next room." Bewildered, Darren and I say a prayer. I drifted back off to sleep.

By September 10th I began to feel human again. Katherine was two days old. The day nurse gave me a sponge bath. It was great! I had not bathed in several days and I was aware that I stunk. I got a new clean and fresh gown. Things were looking up. Darren went and got the breast pump from the NICU. He returned with our digital camera to show me a picture of Katherine. With the nurse's help, they pumped the colostrum from my breasts. Darren kept saying,

"Liquid gold, Tania. Good job!" I was so weak that I could not even hold the pumps to my breasts. The breast-pumping process was repeated several times throughout the day.

Darren and the nurse kept showing me pictures of Katherine to help me bond with her. However, she looked like an alien to me. She was thin and emaciated and she had crazy blond hair. I was in disbelief that she was even mine. I was in denial. When I saw those pictures, I rejected Katherine. She was so small and so frail and perhaps she was not going to make it. I was trying to protect myself.

The nurses asked me if I would like to see my baby that afternoon. They believed I was up to it. Darren was excited. Darren and the nurse hoisted me up. I felt really light-headed and Darren yelled, "Put her down, put her down!" I nearly fainted. I was put back into bed. Perhaps, we would attempt again tomorrow. September 11th was the day I saw Katherine for the first time. She was three days old. The nurse asked me after breakfast if I would like to dangle my feet off of the bed. She explained what she meant and I agreed to try. It felt so good. My incision ached, especially when I pumped my breasts. I was breast pumping by myself now with only occasional assistance from Darren. I felt proud knowing that I was contributing to Katherine's health. Darren brought photos of Katherine to show me. It was my only connection to her. In this latest picture, Katherine wore a mask and had mittens on her hands because she had Jaundice. Darren said she looked like a skier or a boxer. He was always positive, always trying to make me laugh. Poor Darren, he had to go back and forth between the ICU and the NICU to be with his girls.

The catheter was removed. Because I seemed stronger and could now dangle my feet, the nurses encouraged me to go to the washroom by myself. When I stood up and hobbled to the washroom, the nurses gave me a standing ovation. They were very excited for me!

Darren convinced me it was time to meet Katherine later that day. I was very reluctant and nervous. I did not know what to expect. I smiled at Darren. Thank

God for Darren. Darren held the IV stand and off we wheeled to the NICU. When we were in the scrub-in station, Darren explained in lengthy detail how I should wash to limit infecting the NICU with germs. I looked down at my arms. They were bruised and covered by bandages. There were track marks everywhere. An IV lock was sticking out of one hand just in case I required more medications. I washed up as best I could and put on a latex glove covering the IV lock. I really did not know what to expect and was apprehensive. Darren wheeled me to Katherine's bassinet. She was so small, so frail, and so perfect. He encouraged me to touch her but I flatly refused to put my hands anywhere near the bassinet. I thought what if, what if she doesn't make it? What if I fall in love with her and lose her? What if I die myself? I just could not do this. I was upset and emotional. I started to sob. Darren reluctantly took me back to the ICU room at my insistence. Later that same day I was transferred from ICU to the Mother and Baby Ward. I was relieved. It was a welcome refuge because it was very familiar as I had spent most of my hospitalization there.

The next day things were good. I was pumping my breasts like a professional. I had it down to a science. I visualized raindrops on a window beading down to help bring in more milk. It worked. I was up to four baby food jars a pump. There was lots of my milk in the NICU freezer now. I was so proud of myself. I was helping Katherine. I was contributing to her life. I was mothering her. I was seeing Katherine regularly but only when Darren was visiting because I was still confined to a wheelchair. All was well. My IV lock was taken out.

My early afternoon visit with Katherine went better than I could have expected. I watched her breathe. Actually, I was watching her little chest go up and down. I thought to myself, "God, please give me some sort of sign or signal that everything is going to be okay." I held my hand over Katherine and I watched her vitals come down. Katherine sensed it was me. I whispered, "I am here." I reached in further. Suddenly Katherine reached up and grabbed my index finger with her bony little hand and pulled my finger toward her throat. She put my finger on her throat, almost as if to say, "I'm going to be okay, Mom. You don't need to worry about me." I felt my entire body fill with relief. I cannot prove that my blood pressure dropped, but in that moment, my internal vibrating ceased and I relaxed. I kept my hands cupped over her little body for several minutes. I took in deep breaths to the very bottom of my lungs. It was good therapy for both of us.

I walked on my own and showered later that afternoon. It felt awesome to wash my hair. Once more nurses at the nursing station were clapping and cheering me on. I felt such a sense of accomplishment. I was getting better. I was on the mend. I was going to make it. I came back to the room and put on some lip gloss and mascara, blow-dried my hair and then collapsed into bed. This was more activity, in the past forty-five minutes then I had done in weeks! I was exhausted but at least I looked good. Yet, I needed to rest and recover.

I was given my usual medication at the end of the evening. I sensed that the dosage wasn't right but I took it. I was on so much medication, which was constantly adjusted, so it was really hard to stay on top of things. Although it was the same medication, I was given fast rather than slow release. It was a very serious error. My blood pressure dropped so rapidly, I developed chills. I pressed my switch on the bed to call the nurses. I thought I was having a Celiac attack because it felt similar to when I ingest gluten. I felt nauseous, cold and exhausted. The nurses placed warm blankets on me and I collapsed with exhaustion.

Jody, one of my favourite nurses, took my vitals in the morning. I told her about the previous night's crisis. We had a discussion about gluten. I said I was concerned that my food was being cross-contaminated with gluten. Jody assured me that she would order a consultation with the dietician and relay my concerns. Jody asked me to take my medication and when I told her that I took something different last night, she was puzzled. I showed her the medication packets in the garbage and luckily they were still there. She blurted, "Oh my goodness!" When my obstetrician found out what had happened, he was angry with the nurses, and yelled at them. I told him, "It was an accident. No big deal." Later that day blood pressure rocketed to 222/143, well above normal (120/80).

I was transferred to Intensive Care Unit (ICU) for observation. I was once again hooked up on tubes, poked and prodded. I had a blood pressure cuff on my left arm that inflated every ten or fifteen minutes. My obstetrician was livid. He came "flying" into the ICU in his hospital attire just after performing a delivery and yelled at the doctors, "I did my part. I delivered a healthy baby. You get her blood pressure down and get her home with her husband where she belongs!" My blood pressure normalized after a new medication was introduced. It felt like my abdomen became unlocked. I felt relief. I had never noticed it before, but colour became more vibrant as my blood pressure came down. Green became greener and red became redder and so on. Because my blood pressure was elevated for so long, it had affected my perception of colour. During my high blood pressure episodes, I never once suffered the intense headaches that most people did, or potential loss of eyesight. Amazingly I was unaffected and I had more energy than I normally did. My only physical complaint was my neck. It was always stiff when my blood pressure was abnormally high.

Darren was extremely frustrated and angry because of the second trip to the ICU. I was indifferent to it all. I felt fine. I did not really understand the severity of this situation. After all, it is just numbers to me. The chief ICU doctor came and explained to me that I was in the ICU on stroke watch. He went into a lengthy detail about what could happen (e.g. stroke, aneurysm, or blood clots). This was not good, not good at all. In fact, one senior nurse, a nice grey-haired lady, pointed out to Darren that she had never seen blood pressure that high. That was great, just great. "Okay," I say. "Whatever it takes to get out of here, I will do."

I was sent back to the Mother and Baby Ward during the wee hours of the next morning. My blood pressure was stabilized. This latest combination of medications seemed to be working. I climbed back into "my bed" and off to sleep I went. My obstetrician discharged me in the morning and said that I could go home and be with my husband. I was really excited about this. When I phoned Darren, he was in disbelief. What! How can it be that forty-eight hours previously, I was in the intensive care unit on stroke watch and twelve hours later I can go home? I did not care and did not question. I enthusiastically said, "Come and pick me up at lunch time." I fervently packed up my stuff, the suitcase of clothing, the makeup, the hot rollers and the baby gifts. I pumped my breasts again. After I finished pumping, I sat down, chewed on a piece of gum, watched some television and had a nap.

Darren came and hauled all my belongings downstairs using the wheelchair and loaded the car. He insisted that I should not help and said, "Just go and visit Maria," a long-term patient and baby-ward buddy. Darren demanded that I sit in the wheelchair to get wheeled downstairs. Although I told him that I thought it was silly, I sat in it anyway. We went out for lunch together at a local restaurant and then returned to spend the afternoon with Katherine in the NICU. I needed to take several breaks to walk from the parking lot to the elevator, which was less than one city block. I was winded and out of shape. It took every ounce of energy out of me. Darren was understanding and patient.

When Darren and I visited Katherine, I would usually go to a different room and pump my breasts. I would return to visit some more. It always amazed me how much her vitals would even out, level off and become more rhythmic when I returned. The nurses told us that parents who interacted more with their babies in the hospital were also able to get their babies out faster. The nurses encouraged me to bring a picture of Darren and I to put in Katherine's crib so that she could look at us. I knew that babies could only see twelve inches away, but I liked that intention. We brought pictures the next day.

I was so happy to be home at the condo and familiar surroundings. I was back in my own bed and eating what I wanted to eat. I would even get to snuggle with Darren tonight. Yippee! It was two months since I was able to be in bed with my husband. I had a strange dream that night. I was in a tub of balls, like the kind you see at children's play structures, and I was sinking, drowning in them. I awoke screaming "Darren save me, save me!" What could this mean?
I had trouble settling down to sleep but Darren comforted me and we both drifted off to sleep again.

I felt that all was well. Katherine was progressing nicely. She was only on the ventilator one day and the Jaundice was gone. There was no brain bleeding, which I was told are common in premature babies. She was gaining weight sufficiently. The NICU doctors were calling her a star! I would be able to hold her when she was about three pounds. I was so excited and looking forward to that experience. I had conflicting emotions the day that I was to hold Katherine. I was really excited and full of sweet anticipation. However, when I was holding her, I had a thought, "What would happen if I threw her up against the wall? I bet she would die." Where the hell did that come from? I was horrified! I said to that voice inside my head, "Stop" and it went away. I never shared that thought with Darren or anyone else until I joined the Postpartum Support Group at the YMCA where I felt safe enough to utter those words. I was ashamed that I could think something so horrible. Moms are not supposed to think things like that. Moms are supposed to be filled with positive thoughts, energy and emotions.

Over the next week I was in a routine where I would wake up and take my medications, eat, shower and then go and visit Katherine. The doctor's did their rounds in the mornings, so you could not go to the NICU until after they were finished. Sometimes, I would go in the hospital and visit my mother-in-law, Linda, and have a cup of tea. Then I would go to the NICU and spend the afternoon with Katherine.

I kept thinking that it would be great if Darren could take paternity leave. His salary would get topped up to 95% for the year. I could just do my Mary Kay cosmetic business full-time, an entrepreneurial activity that I have been doing since 2000. This way we could be together as a family and have the best of everything. We'd have enough money and family time. I started to obsess about this thought. Also, I was finding excuses to not go and see as much of Katherine as I should have. I told myself that the doctors were doing rounds in the morning, so I could not go then. Darren and I would be going in the evening so why bother going in the afternoon as well.

I started obsessing about Mary Kay. I couldn't get the obsessive thoughts out of my head. They played over and over again in my mind. I thought I should be doing Mary Kay full-time. I needed to become a Director so that I could stay home. I needed to make enough money so that I didn't have to return to work at SaskTel. Mary Kay Directors were always saying to become Directors quickly. My priorities were changing. My focus was on my career instead of Katherine. This was very obsessive behaviour. I was sliding out of control.

I was writing constantly in my journal about women that I knew I wanted to have on my Mary Kay team. I even phoned my Mary Kay Director and told her my plans. Of course, she was thrilled. I don't believe she realized that I switched my focus from Katherine to my Mary Kay team members and that it was consuming my life. I would go over to her house and share my lists of potential team members and activities I had planned. I called my customers to tell them I decided to pursue Mary Kay full-time and asked them to be part of my team. I was calling some people at six or seven in the morning. I was a woman on a mission! I justified my behaviour to myself and to Darren. I rationalized that not visiting Katherine was okay because self-employment meant that I would be able to work from home, permanently. Reflecting back, this was the first trigger that something was really going awry.

About three days after I was discharged from the hospital, I began having troubles sleeping. I was restless and tossed and turned all night. I had little control over my thoughts. I was looking for meaning in my life and wanted answers to life questions. "Why did this crisis happen to me? What was my purpose in life?" I felt that I had been given a second chance. There had to be more to this. I would lie in bed and stew for hours. Darren was exhausted and would nod off to sleep. I assumed that he thought I was sleeping too. I could not calm my mind down. It would spiral and spiral like a snowball rolling down a hill, one thought after another after another. I would get up and pump my breasts. It distracted me for a short while. Then I would try lying down again; toss, turn, turn and toss. Argh ... Okay, maybe a hot bath. Into the tub – no, that did not help either. Nothing would stop my mind from the racing thoughts.

I literally did not sleep for the next three days. I was delusional. I could not shut off my mind. I remember the evening of September 21st, going to bed and thinking about all the terrible stuff going on in the world; wars, starving people, neglect, greed, fear, rape, etc. I could not get it out of my mind. Why, why, why? As I searched for meaning, I had an epiphany. Hey, if money, (what I really meant was fear and greed) did not matter, the world would become peaceful and right itself. If money had no real value and there were no stock exchanges, then people would not be concerned about money. People would work at jobs they loved and the world would be transformed. It was at that moment that I saw the world from far away, like a picture you would see in National Geographic, in my mind's eye and it exploded. It was a revelation. I have to act, I thought. I wanted to raise Katherine in a better world; a world free from pain and suffering. Hysteria was setting in.

The next morning I got up around 5 am and went to the television. I prayed, "Dear God, give me a sign." I turned on the television and saw a rainbow and the sun rising. There was nothing negative broadcasting on television. I mean it, nothing! The 6:00 am news cast reported only positive information. A plane had successfully landed after all the passengers started praying. There was nothing of significance reported about the stock markets, and a sacred statue of five women from different cultures was discovered. This was my sign. To this day, I don't know if these events occurred or were figments of my imagination. I quietly dressed and snuck out of the condo. Darren was still fast asleep. It was 6:30 in the morning. I felt inspired. I was going to change the world.

I went over to my Mary Kay director's house, which was only five houses from our condo. Nancy was in her bathrobe drinking a cup of tea. I was so excited, perhaps even manic. I told her that we women were going to heal the world and that if money didn't matter, the world would fix itself. I thought I was making complete sense. Nancy was smiling and nodding. I told her I was having a conversation with God. I saw signs everywhere. "Look!" I pointed to the television in the kitchen, "That guy is going to be our Prime Minister." It was Stephen Harper who did become Prime Minister later that year. I hugged

Nancy, when I said good-bye and off I left. I was feeling quite empowered.

I got in the car and thought, "Now what?" Action was required. Yes, a female anchorwoman was required to interview the Pope. The Pope would help with the politicians and explain how we could soothe and calm Mother Earth by getting rid of stock markets and currency. I drove to a local television building. I felt that a recognizable local anchorwoman at the time could help me with this endeavour. I went to the building and asked to speak to her. They told me she was not in so I asked if I could borrow their computer and compose a letter. They agreed. I sat at the front reception computer and poured my heart out on paper. I then pulled out a Mary Kay autobiography book and the letter I had just typed and asked that they give them to the anchorwoman. She would know what to do.

I felt quite pleased with myself. I was going to go home but before I did, I was going to see Katherine. She would be so proud of her mommy. I was fixing the world. I sat with Katherine until rounds started at 9:00 am. I drove home and was planning to tell Darren that I was going to immediately quit my full-time job. He could take full paternity leave. Wouldn't that be exciting! When I walked into the condo, Darren was awake and looked really worried. He told me we were going to go for a drive. I readily went with him to the car. We chit-chatted and I asked where we were going. Darren told me the hospital. I thought to myself, "How nice, we will get to see Katherine again."

Darren pulled into the emergency entrance to the hospital. I thought this was strange but I did not comment. We walked in together holding hands. Again, the admitting staff knew my name, "Tania we have been expecting you." "You have," I thought. We were met by a psychiatrist who introduced himself as a psychiatrist. He took us to a nicely decorated room. Darren asked me to tell the psychiatrist the thoughts I was having. I told him that I wanted to heal the world, make money with Mary Kay, quit my job full-time job at SaskTel, and that I was having regular conversations with God. The psychiatrist looked at me in disbelief. He then told me that he wanted me to stay at the hospital for observation. I agreed because I thought I'd be closer to Katherine.

I was admitted to the Psychiatric Ward and told that I would have to take a high dose of anti-psychotic drugs. I was agreeable with taking medication until they told me that I would be unable to give Katherine anymore of my breast milk because it could transfer through my milk to her. "What? How dare they?" Darren and I had an argument. I threatened divorce. I knew this would cut him to the core. "How dare he? I was fine!" When I look back at this argument, it has been the only argument I have ever had with Darren where I threatened divorce. Darren did not appear to be crushed by my comments. He looked me calmly in the eye and said "Fine, just get better." Pure love was in his eyes. He was not malicious. He was not callous. He showed genuine concern and love for me.

Reluctantly, I swallowed the damn pill and I crashed hard. I slept, and slept, and slept. Within a couple of days, that sense of internal vibration from the inside left. The vibrating felt like someone was grabbing my arteries and dangling them like puppets on a string. I could finally sleep. I could think, but I was having difficulty counting when we would play cribbage. My mind was tricking me. In retrospect, I believe it was the combination of sleep deprivation and the medication that led to difficulties with concentration. For example, I could swear that I saw a wedding band on my father-in-law's left hand. It was his Saskatchewan Roughrider football alumni ring. I thought I would see people enter an entranceway and then vanish. My mind was playing tricks on me. I thought I was going crazy! Two plus two was not adding properly. It was really frustrating. I would say to my head "Go away and leave me alone." Finally, reality became reality, after several days of sleeping through the night.

I stayed in the Psychiatric Ward for two weeks in total. My parents came to visit. Darren came to visit. Everyone wanted me to get better. I wanted to get better. I got out several times on day passes for good behaviour and was allowed to stay overnight with my husband at the condo. During my psychiatric stay, I was allowed to visit Katherine at my leisure so long as I signed out at the nurse's station. I was discharged on October 3rd and visited Katherine every opportunity I had until she was discharged from the NICU three and a half weeks later. The whole ordeal of the psychiatric stay shook me to my core. I hadn't recognized that I was even sick. I would not accept it. I had felt fine and I was extremely happy before being taken to the hospital. In fact, on a scale of one to ten, I was at least a fourteen in terms of happiness and joy. So, when I took the medication to correct that manic feeling, it made me feel vulnerable. I had to re-assess my mental state. I felt incompetent as a mother and was reluctant to be at home with Katherine by myself. I was consumed with doubt and insecurity.

My sister, Kim, came to visit from Edmonton for ten days so that I would not be alone with Katherine. Darren returned to work because he couldn't afford to take any more time off. I welcomed my sister. I willingly let Kim cuddle and snuggle Katherine. I felt so inferior to my sister. I felt useless as a mom. I felt that Kim was doing a better job than ever I could with Katherine. These feelings only intensified as Kim's ten-day stay came to a close. Kim would ask me questions like, "Do you feel bonded to the baby?" What did that mean? I didn't know. I would always answer, "Yes." I was withdrawn and not my usual, talkative and open self. The anti-psychotic medication made me tired and sleepy. It even sucked away my libido. I had no energy, no gusto, and no motivation. I was on a downward spiral and I didn't know how to help myself.

I had extreme difficulties getting out of bed if I did not have something planned in the morning. I literally could just stay in my pajamas all day and lie in bed with Katherine. I never made supper, did the laundry or cleaned the condo. I could barely take a shower myself. I never put on makeup and I just tossed my hair into a ponytail. This is very uncharacteristic of me. I usually had pride in my appearance. I am not even sure if I brushed my teeth every day.

Darren would feed the baby in the morning, get showered and dressed, eat, and then wake me when he went to work. When he came home, he made supper, did laundry, took care of Katherine and conducted the feeding in the middle of the night. This routine continued until Katherine was ten months old. I don't know how he did it. He really deserved "Husband and Father of the Year" awards. He never complained to me. He was forever supportive. He was my rock.

I joined Sally Elliott's Postpartum Support Group at the YMCA about one month after my sister went home. It was good to be with other women who were having the same problems. We all could relate to each other. We shared laughter and tears. It was there that I met Cheryl who told me about a Wednesday morning Bible discussion study with Gloria (www.tapestryministries.ca). That sounded good. "What the heck....I'll try it." I went to it and really enjoyed it. They had a babysitting service so I knew Katherine was in capable hands. It was good to have a short break from Katherine. It was there that I met friendly faces and smiles. No one knew the turmoil or Hell I was experiencing. I would smile and be pleasant but I was screaming inside. I was wearing the mask!

Turn the page or skip this paragraph if you are suffering with depression right now. The following information may be too graphic and not help your situation. I was not suicidal but I thought about it a lot. I had obsessive thoughts about dying. I wanted to kill Katherine, Darren and myself. I would think of creative ways to murder Darren. I rationalized that it had to be while he was sleeping because he was bigger and stronger. I was in a world of pain. I remember sometimes phoning Darren at work and saying things like "I know how I am going to do it." Darren would calmly talk to me, hang up the phone and then phone one of my girlfriends, my mom, cousins or sisters. He'd say things like, "Tania could use some company. Could you go over there this afternoon?" Darren never told any of them about the negative thoughts I was having. I felt safe with Darren. That is why I shared those awful thoughts with him. If you talk about it, it has less power over you. Deep down I knew I needed to talk. This must have been a huge burden on Darren's already laden-down shoulders. As I write this paragraph, I truly hope that I can save someone's life. You are not alone! I feel sad, that my mom or grandma or sister may read this, but it is truth and truth sets all free. Nobody explained to me that taking the anti-psychotic medication would make me into a zombie. I was numb. I really did not feel emotion. I felt like a shell, looking nice on the outside, but hollow on the inside. Another side effect of the medication was cravings for fattening foods. I don't really like peanut butter but I would eat it by the tablespoon full, and eat one-kilogram container every week. It's no wonder that I never lost the baby weight. In fact, when I started Weight Watchers in the Fall, after returning to work, I weighed a whopping 205 pounds, yikes. As well, the medication blocked my libido. I had none. It was non-existent. I have never in my life experienced this before. I love snuggling, holding hands, kissing, and sex. All of a sudden, it was gone. This put an additional strain on my relationship with Darren because until this point, our sex life had been fantastic. To further add insult to injury, my blood pressure was still so high that any kind of physical activity, including sex, scared me. I was able to walk a couple of kilometers but it made me ill. I was physically out of shape.

Luckily for me, my mom would come over on Monday mornings for breakfast and force me to get up. She would make breakfast and take care of Katherine while I took a shower. Darren's father co-coordinated a weekly breakfast date with me on Thursday mornings at 9:00 am sharp. I remember one time going to the hotel for our breakfast date, looking awful. My hair was not done. I wore sweats and didn't do my hair or make-up. Larry said to me, "This is a date. Next week you better have your hair and makeup done." That was really good for me to hear because it helped me to change my behaviour and recognize that I was depressed.

I would meet my girlfriends from the Postpartum Support Group for coffee or a walk around Wascana Lake in addition to our weekly meetings on Wednesdays. I would also meet my "normal" girlfriends who were on maternity leave for coffee on Friday mornings. No one ever asked about my Postpartum Depression, but they knew. I was very appreciative that they planned the get-togethers early in the day. They knew I would not get out bed otherwise.

I kept to a routine as much as possible. I did not like being alone with Katherine because I would have stupid thoughts. I am just going to say that I could have given Stephen King a run for his money. Bathing, feedings and time alone with Katherine were difficult. When I was alone with her, I would read Sandra Boynton books because they rhymed. It took my mind off of the awful thoughts and the intentions to harm Katherine and myself. I would read and re-read the books for hours on end.

I would count down the hours until Darren would come home from work so that I could have a break and not feel that Katherine was one hundred percent dependent on me. I resented the fact that someone could be so totally reliant on me, especially someone who was so helpless and vulnerable. I told Darren how her dependency made me feel. He would say, "What did you think parenting was going to be about?" This made me feel worse because I should have known better and suffered with more guilt. I have a sister, Shirrae, who is thirteen years younger than me, so I have had experience looking after a young child and know the reliance they have on adults. In retrospect, my feelings included anger, resentment, frustration, guilt, and rage, to say the least. I knew in my heart of hearts, that this feeling of inadequacy, anger and resentment was not right. Parenting was not supposed to be like this!

I learned how to cope with my negative feelings through talking to other mothers, reading self-help books (The Secret and You Can Heal Your Life were two of my favourites),[2] listening to feel-good music, and continually reminding myself that "this too shall pass." Praying and reading the Bible were comforting to me. Journaling, seeking therapy and going back to work all helped me regain my sanity.

The inspirational quote, "You cannot change the wind, but you can change your sail" really speaks to this valley of my life. I feel that we can't let the adversity prevent us from living. Instead, we need to look for ways to heal ourselves. I take comfort in knowing that life is ebbs and flows, ups and downs, peaks and valleys. I think that the saying "this too shall pass" eventually comes true. I also believe that in order to experience love and truly appreciate the feeling of love, you have to experience hate. Emotions have opposites, just like day and night. You flip back and forth. I am grateful to have experienced all of these emotions because it has helped me to grow into the person I am today.

I started to appreciate Katherine when she was ten months old. I could relax when I was with her. I loved spending time with her, instead of dreading the hours alone and counting down until Darren came home. I was healing. I was also upset that in eight short weeks, I would be returning to work. How unfair it all seemed. I was finally feeling "right," and like a mom should feel. I considered this to be my time of feeling bonded to Katherine. It finally happened and I understood what my sister, Kim, was asking me eight months ago.

I went back to work mid September. The distraction was good. I was in my comfort-zone again. I felt competent. At work I got to see and catch up with people I had not seen in over a year. Katherine was at the YMCA Day Care and was well looked after. Life was on track.

I continued to see my psychiatrist and every visit it would be the same request. I requested to get off the anti-psychotic medication because I knew I was not my true self. The doses were decreased slowly. I was also seeing a psychologist about my feelings about being a poor mother, and anger, depression and rage. I always asked her, "How do you know if you are being a good mom?" She would always say things like, "Tell me about Katherine. Is she growing, thriving and reaching developmental milestones? Children who are unloved and neglected don't do these things - they regress or show physical, behavioural or developmental delays." My child was excelling. The hospital tracks the child for the first three years of their life when they were in the NICU. They send you quarterly assessments for you to complete. This is great because I received information on developmental milestones, something some parents don't know about. It was good. I like this information. As a proud parent, I can tell you with confidence that Katherine is exceeding expectations in all areas; physical, mental, and emotional.

Darren and I also went to marriage counselling. It seemed to me, the better I got, the worse Darren got. He was angry, frustrated and miserable. It was difficult to live with him. I think he was finally able to show his emotions now that the crisis was over. It wasn't a fun home life for either of us. Sex was almost non-existent and when it did occur, I was resentful. Our psychologist helped Darren and I focus on the good in our relationship and the bonding we felt when I was hospitalized which ultimately lead to forgiveness. I forgave. Darren forgave. I slowly and completely weaned off Olazaphine, or as I fondly nick-named it "fat-opine," because of the weight gain it caused, by February 2007. We gelled as a cohesive family unit on our three-week vacation to Maui, Hawaii the same month. I am so grateful for that experience.

Looking back over the last three years, I am thankful to have had this experience. I hope that sharing my story will help many women and families. It is really our collective truths, Carla, Elita and our husbands. I truly believe that Postpartum Depression is more common than the statistics indicate. I believe there is a spectrum of postpartum difficulties. When I talk to women more often than not, they comment about either their own personal experiences or they know someone who has suffered, too. This epidemic needs to be talked about so that women can take their power back. I believe that communities can provide more support and encouragement. Women with Postpartum Depression, you are not alone. We are all one through energy and being on Earth together. It is our responsibility to assist each other; after all, we each have two hands, one hand to help ourselves, one hand to help others.

I have deeper and more meaningful relationships since suffering from PPD and psychosis. I have a sense of calm and confidence that I never had prior and I feel purpose for my life. I have forgiven other people's transgressions as well as my own. I experience abundance and gratitude every day.

Chapter Four

The Husbands' Perspectives

Peggy Collins

The best way out is always through.

~ Robert Frost

❝ Who are we to judge? Do we understand the whole picture? What is the truth? Supporting someone who is experiencing mental illness is an unbelievable challenge. How do people do it? What is it like for those who are closest to them? What is it like for the husbands of wives who are suffering from Postpartum Depression?" I talked with the three men involved in the previous stories, and I can tell you with all honesty, it can be "Hell on Earth."

It is important to represent these men and what they have to say. Most often, in cases like these, the attention is directed mostly at the patients with the illness, the mothers. The husbands' stories will help other men. My wish is that this chapter will catch the attention of men who face this daunting challenge. My hope is to inspire them to not give up and to cheer them on; to provide them insight on how other husbands managed their way through such adversity, and to give them hope!

It may even be useful information for men who are contemplating fatherhood. He could learn about potential signs of Postpartum Depression symptoms. He could gain insight into the experience of pregnancy, childbirth and child care from a husbands' perspective. He could gain an appreciation of what it takes to hold a marriage together even when the odds are against you.

This chapter could also shed some insight for women. As explained in the book "Men are from Mars and Women are from Venus," by John Gray, Ph.D., men often think and approach situations differently than women. It's important to note that these husbands cared deeply about their loved ones throughout their ordeal, and showed it in their own ways. They were somewhat misunderstood by their wives and others.

I would like to introduce Curtis, Ward and Darren. They are all married to women who have gone through varying degrees of Postpartum Depression. As described in the women's individual stories, their illness nearly destroyed their family relationships. Somehow these men found the courage to hang in there; they found ways to cope and believed that the nightmare they were living would end.

I wanted to know what it was like for them. Were there signs? Were they prepared for the illness that overcame their lives, and if not, how did they gain more knowledge? How did they support their wife and child? Did they get help from others? I wanted to know how the circumstances affected them personally, their jobs, and their health. Did the experience change their perspective on life? Did it make them stronger people? And of course, what advice could they offer other men going through similar experiences. I interviewed each husband separately. Amazingly, I was hearing almost the same story from all three. They suffered the same grief, challenges and shared common coping skills.

It was painful, demoralizing, disappointing, draining and frightening. These are some of the emotions Curtis, Ward and Darren collectively experienced. They all said they were afraid to go to work, terrified that they would come home to find their baby or wife or both dead. They were afraid to sleep through the night fearing that their baby or even they themselves would be harmed. There were times when they were totally frustrated. Their households were left in turmoil each day and their basic needs were not being met. Ward and Darren admitted that their anger was so great, at times, that they nearly became physically abusive towards their spouses. Thank God they were able to control such impulses and behaviours. It was all so hard to understand. They would ask themselves over and over why their wives would not just get up, get the help they needed and solve their problems. It was almost impossible for them to comprehend their wives' situation. They knew it wasn't easy for their wives, but sometimes the situation seemed all but hopeless. Their only solace, at times, was turning to alcohol to numb the pain.

Their lives are much calmer now. They have weathered the storm and have found a greater sense of peace. For the most part, their relationships are mending as the women's stories are being expressed. Of course they still have the battle scars and still need to heal and grow, but they now envision hope for the future and prosperity as a family. They are stronger because of the experiences and they developed maturity and tolerance beyond their ages.

Curtis's Truth

To see Curtis and Carla's wedding pictures you would swear they were models in a wedding magazine. Everything was perfect and beautiful. They were full of hope and promise. Little did they know what was "in store" for them. Out of the three families described in this book, their story, I believe, holds the most heart wrenching long term effects of Postpartum Depression on their lives and their experiences with parenthood. They struggled for over four years with Carla's severe Postpartum Psychosis and Obsessive Compulsive Disorder. Their story is fascinating but cruel. Yet, at the same time, it is very inspiring. One can learn that Curtis' perspective of never giving up hope, really works!

Everything about Carla's pregnancy seemed normal. She and Curtis were both very excited and went through the joyful time of picking out clothes, colours for walls and even names for their expectant new arrival. They briefly heard of Postpartum Depression in pre-natal class, but never for a second believed anything like that could happen to them. All was going along so smoothly. That is except when Carla's best friend's baby died. He was stillborn at about thirty-three weeks along in the pregnancy. The two women were friends going through this wonderful time of childbirth and expectant parenthood together. They had all kinds of dreams and aspirations. This tragic event affected Carla greatly. Carla felt that her friend's loss gave her an unfair advantage in life because she still had her baby growing beautifully inside of her. Carla was consumed with guilt about the whole issue and also worried that perhaps her baby would die too. All this negative anxiety may or may not have contributed to what Carla and Curtis were about to experience. One can only speculate that it did.

Curtis was also greatly saddened by their friend's loss and was at the couple's side along with Carla to provide them support. Oddly enough though, Curtis didn't really see the full impact the death of their friend's baby was having on Carla. There weren't any behaviours that would alert Curtis of what was going on inside of Carla's mind and spirit. Many of us are very good at hiding our emotions. The impact of such behaviour can be devastating. According to Curtis, Carla did have a tendency to obsessively worry about things. Perhaps this made her more vulnerable to Postpartum Depression. Again, one can only speculate.

Cameron, their healthy baby boy, was born on November 17, 2003. He was perfect! Carla was not! It all began twenty-four hours after Cameron's birth. Carla had a terrifying dream that the nurses gave her Cameron, but he was dead. She was shaken, crying and very distressed. She slept only a little for the next few days. She was in physical pain and also had difficulty breastfeeding. But far worse than that, were the horrible voices and visions. Carla heard voices telling her to smother her baby and visions to hurt him. Something was seriously wrong and little Cameron was only two days old. It was Postpartum Psychosis.

When Carla finally shared what was going on with Curtis, he was in absolute shock. Curtis had never even heard of the baby blues never mind Postpartum Depression. He didn't panic but rather felt numb all over. "I am the kind of guy who accepts what's happening and just carries on making the best of it," said Curtis. There were no warning signs at anytime along this journey. How could this have happened to them? "We were so happy and elated with our new baby, but that happiness was short lived," recalls Curtis. "I assumed this would be a short thing – that there had to be a light at the end of the tunnel. It's not a train." He never imagined that he really was dealing with a train and that it was about to turn his life upside down.

"All I could think about was how much this sucked and how disappointing it was. I approached it with a head-down mentality. I had to find a way to fix it. But of course there is very little I could do other than provide support and be strong for Carla and Cameron. There are no quick fixes for Postpartum Psychosis, only ways to cope and somehow make it easier." For Curtis that meant he had to adopt a "toughen up" mentality. "Someone is going to hurt and someone is going to have to carry the weight," stated Curtis. "I needed to accept that weight and do what I had to do to get through this."

Curtis talked about how he came to the realization that his family had a new "normal" now. They had to focus on one day at a time. Carla had difficulty being alone with Cameron, even though she cared for him every day when Curtis was at work. It was at night when Carla had the most difficulty. She loved Cameron deeply but she worried that she would hurt him. All this put a lot of stress and worry on Curtis' shoulders. He would come home from work and not know what to expect. Would his family be alright? Would his son still be safe or even alive? There was also suicide to worry about. It was a terrifying and disturbing time. "I'd rather meet a grizzly bear in a campground, than deal with this. At least the bear is something tangible. How do you solve such an intangible problem as mental illness? There wasn't much I could do."

Carla was receiving help from psychologists and doctors. It wasn't helping much. "During one such visit the doctor told me that Carla's condition would improve very little if any at all, and that I should think about getting a divorce. It was devastating to hear, but I knew that I could not go through with that. I had to stick by Carla and carry out my duties as a husband and father," Curtis said with a determined look on his face.

Curtis was traumatized. The stress was obviously wearing him down. "I was having trouble getting completely relaxed. There was always a feeling of tension in my body, like a constant fear of impending doom," Curtis described what it was like for him. "The constant stress raised my sensitivity to other perceived threats. I would worry more about things like the safety of Cameron in everyday non-threatening situations, like riding his bike or going to the park. You get sensitized to always be on alert – it wears you out."

It has been over four long years of "warfare" for Curtis. He reflected on a statement made by one of the nurses in the hospital a few days after Cameron was born and Carla's condition was diagnosed. "The breastfeeding was not going well. We were all stressed out about it. Cameron was screaming from frustration and hunger. Carla was in tears. I demanded that someone bring us a bottle with formula so that we could solve this problem. When Cameron drank the formula and felt better, I was elated. The nurse looked at me and warned me not to get too happy; there was a huge challenge lurking ahead of us. She was trying to prepare us for the truck that was about to hit – a truck we had no idea how to deal with. Maybe ignorance was bliss." This conversation made Curtis reflect deeply resulting with a tear in his eye.

Curtis' advice for fathers dealing with Postpartum Depression or fathers in general, is to be open to taking on more of the responsibility of parenthood. He even suggested that fathers should take the paternity time if offered by his employer. "We can't just leave it to the mothers to carry the load, especially when dealing with mental illnesses. You can't gamble with your child's life. It's important to talk to people about what is going on and get the help you need. It is important to be a part of the pre-natal experience and ask questions about the total picture including Postpartum Depression. It is okay to be who we are and what we need to become to succeed. Remember we are not all living the 'Cosby Show.' Things are not always that easy."

Carla and Curtis story is one of triumph over tremendous adversity. Carla is much better. She is completely free of all medications. Curtis senses that Carla has changed since the mental "warfare" in her mind became calmer as she shared her story. Her self-confidence has blossomed. Cameron is a happy-go-lucky, bright little boy, full of promise. The horrible secret and difficult illness that plagued their lives is under control and Curtis believes they are much stronger people for going through it. "We should not take anything for granted and we should appreciate our lives and the people we share them with."

Even though Carla and Curtis were able to overcome the challenges of a mental illness in their family, their marriage was weakened. There was simply too much pain and heartache. The stress of dealing with the extreme pressure of Postpartum Depression had taken its toll on their relationship. In 2008, Curtis and Carla decided to divorce but remain amicable friends and co-parents.

Ward's Truth

When little Ella came into this world on March 13th, 2006, Ward and Elita never imagined how dramatically their lives would change. Of course, everyone knows that people's lives are never the same after bringing a child into the world, but they weren't expecting their parenting experience to be so challenging for the first two years. What stands out most for Ward are the memories of Ella's endless crying and the extreme anxiety that Elita was experiencing. It was total chaos. Ella was colicky and cried out in pain much of the time. There were also problems with breastfeeding and Elita was obviously not doing very well emotionally. She wasn't sleeping much; she became paranoid about everything, even to leave the house.

Ward had some advice for the men out there. "Women definitely change after childbirth. Men should be prepared for that. They are not the same women we marry. Of course it is a bit more dramatic of a change when Postpartum Depression symptoms are present. It's difficult at first to determine whether what you are going through is normal stress of parenthood, or is there more to this situation. It would be easier to sort through it when or if you had a second child. When you have your first child you have nothing to compare it to, so you don't know what is right or normal."

"It seemed that Elita was losing her patience with Ella more than you would normally expect. I too would get frustrated with all the demands she made on us, and sometimes get angry. However, Elita was very intense. She often yelled hysterically. Postpartum Depression heightened her anxiety and she had few coping skills. The level of stress was alarming. It felt like our family was going to collapse. I remember thinking that if this doesn't straighten out soon I don't know what the 'Hell' I'm going to do. I was not prepared to give up on Elita, but I knew we needed help. Elita recognized that as well."

Ward truly believed in and acknowledged Elita's love for Ella. "She adores her daughter," he said. He also believes that there is an element of independence about Ella that doesn't completely fulfill Elita's needs as a mother. "Ella isn't an overly affectionate child. She doesn't really like to be cuddled, which is what Elita craved. I know this added to Elita's anxiety." Ward openly praises Ella's independence. He sees the benefits as it pertains to her ability to be confident and true to herself. He also knows that Elita believes in these benefits, but it is obvious that Elita still has a desire to experience the softer side of raising a child.

When Ward and Elita were learning about pregnancy and childbirth, they were introduced to the possibility of Postpartum Depression. In the back of Ward's mind he did wonder if this could happen to them. Elita suffered with heightened anxiety and was somewhat lacking self-confidence before she became pregnant. Yet, she really had no reason to not feel good about herself. Ward has seen her excel and achieve many goals in her life. Lacking self-confidence combined with anxiety are two precursors to the illness. He said that he was not totally surprised when she developed Postpartum Depression. He also noticed that Elita seemed better than ever since writing this book. Her outgoing confident personality and her positive self-perception, is even better than before Ella was born.

Ward felt that they still lacked information about thorough parenting skills, even though they went through all the pre-natal education that's generally available. Actual parenting education was only touched on in class. He recognized that there is so much to know and so much to search through to see what really works, (e.g. deciding when a baby should and should not sleep). It became

138

apparent to Ward and Elita that they should just let Ella sleep when she wanted and needed. Ella was a lot less cranky and much easier to deal with once they discovered this concept.

Ward began to look for ways to cope during the height of the turmoil. The stress was severe. He would get calls at work from Elita where she tearfully expressed her anxiety and despair. As soon as he got home from work, she handed him a crying baby. Elita could not handle any more time caring for Ella. She would be in her pajamas all day and did little around the house. The majority of her days were spent cooped up inside her home. She rarely left her surroundings. The situation seemed hopeless. Ward reflected, "I wasn't sure that I wanted to be around my family much. I worked more than I needed to. I know that I was using work as a coping mechanism. I even drank more than I usually would. It was a very difficult time and I became sick of it. Resentment was setting in."

"I just wanted Elita to get up and get some help. Go talk to people, and find a support group. Admitting that there was a problem and searching for a solution would only make me think more highly of Elita not less, which I believe was the opposite of what she thought."

This is an amazing perception that is worth exploring. I believe most women are afraid to show their vulnerabilities or perceived weaknesses to the men in their lives. Yet, all three of the men said that they would look up to their wives more if she would have acknowledged that there was a problem, tried to solve it by getting help and address the problem head-on. It was more disappointing for them to see their wives become victims of the situation, therefore manifesting a "poor me" attitude and feeling shame. I also believe that women with Postpartum Depression are frightened and shamed by the symptoms, so they try to hide them. It is the nature of the illness.

Ward noticed some symptoms that could have been indications of Postpartum Depression. Elita was not comfortable being left alone with Ella, especially for long periods of time. There was definitely a loving bond between Elita and Ella, but at times this bond seemed forced. Parenting did not appear to come naturally. This became apparent when watching them play. Elita seemed uncomfortable at times. She was just going through the motions and would often mirror how Ward would play with Ella.

Another symptom was that Elita lost interest in maintaining a regular daily routine or caring about her appearance. She seemed to lose interest in her own well being. It was almost as if she became paralyzed and unmotivated with life itself. Although Ward believes that getting up and out of the house with a daily routine could greatly improve the situation, in his opinion, Elita just didn't see that as a solution. Ward recommended that if husbands or others in the family are seeing these behaviours, they should confront the situation with their wives in a compassionate way and seek help from Family Physicians, Mental Health professionals and support groups.

"As well, find someone like a close friend to confide in, even better if it's someone who is going through a similar situation to yours. Having a close friend like that was a saving grace for me. It's important to spend time with buddies that you can bond with and talk about your experiences. A good laugh never hurts either, even if it's at your wife's expense," as Ward chuckles. Alone time was also helpful to Ward. "If you want to get out of the house for awhile, be sure to set up a babysitter, so that your wife has some time for herself as well. Believe me you'll be happy you did."

Husbands have to carry a fair share of responsibility and emotional stress, and it can become exhausting. "It's fine to give all this advice, says Ward, but I found that I was wearing thin and patience was difficult to find some days. It may be hard to see what the right solution is and remain objective and caring. All I can say is get help in any way you can."

Ward admitted that he did not realize how serious the problem really was at the time. It was difficult to know whether to take charge or not, and if he should force his wife to get help. "It's important for the husband to seek advice not only to help his wife, but to get help with his own sanity. There were times when I thought I was going crazy, repeating the same things over and over, trying to solve the same problems. Elita seemed to put up a wall and wouldn't let me empathize with her. She made it known that she was the victim here and I couldn't possibly understand what she was going through. This was very frustrating and I felt angry," Ward reflected on the toughest times of dealing with PPD. He recognized the importance in caring for ourselves first and encourages all mothers in this way. "We can't live our lives in fear of disappointing those around us. We have to be individuals and become the best we can. It has a direct impact on everyone and the success of the family. It comes down to trust and believing that the husband can understand and accept the situation, and to not discount the husbands' ability to help. It also comes down to believing in one's own strength."

The Paterson's are now seeing hope amidst the despair. In some ways, Ward feels that the ordeal that they have lived through has helped their relationship. They have gained a better understanding of themselves and each other. Their communication is more open and they feel that they can rely on each other. "If anything," Ward said with a smile, "It has given us an opportunity to grow as individuals and made for an interesting life." He went on to say that their experiences have created great stories and have even added some humour to help cope. They can laugh at the way they reacted to some of the situations.

"The emotional trials we feel as a parent and a partner has to be a natural part of life. There's no other explanation. It can make you stronger or tear you apart. For us, it made us more motivated to live our ideals and values. It's all a work in progress and I'm not willing to give up on that." Ward's advice for other husbands is to encourage bringing the truth out in the open. "Help your wife see past the mask and be there to support her. You'll likely see it more clearly than she does. Your family is at stake. Ensure she knows that its okay to get the help she needs. Deal with the problem together." Overall his message is to address the problem, instead of running from it. Face the storm head-on. "It's not going away unless you deal with it. The work is worth it because, in our case at least, it has started to lead to a more rewarding and fun-filled life."

Darren's Truth

arren and Tania were both very excited at how quickly they were able to conceive after deciding to start a family. They were at an ideal age to start on this path. Both were in their 30's and both had great jobs. It was like a fairytale. But it wasn't a fairytale. Their lives came crashing down around them. Their vision of happiness turned into a frightening and disappointing ordeal. There was a tremendous amount of stress and trauma prior to the birth of their daughter, Katherine. Tania had severe health problems, with high blood pressure and anxiety. She nearly died twice during her pregnancy. She was heavily medicated over several months both before and after giving birth in an effort to stabilize her medical condition. Katherine was born pre-mature only weighing 2 pounds, 16 ounces. There was a time when both Darren's wife and baby were in Intensive Care, both fighting for their lives at the same time. He spent countless hours watching over them. It was exhausting.

Tania was discharged around ten days after Katherine was born and now home. She displayed bizarre bahaviours that soon led to a complete breakdown in reality. Red flags were everywhere. She didn't sleep for several days. Darren saw that his wife's exuberant personality was suddenly magnified tenfold. There was a definite change in her demeanor and behaviour. Her speech was very disjointed and she rattled on and on about things that made little to no sense. Tania normally kept a very neat and tidy household, but things were in chaos. The house looked like a robber had ransacked it. She would not make any attempts to prepare meals or other household responsibilities. She talked about quitting her full-time job and expanding a home-based business. She visited people around the city, talking erratically and out of character. Darren worried that people would judge her incorrectly, and that she would embarrass herself to the point of losing credibility. Thank goodness that her friends and family recognized the problem and contacted Darren.

Because another family member also had a mental health illness, Darren recognized the signs. "People struggling with mental health breakdown will grasp at anything to emotionally attach to, no matter how blown out of proportion or unrealistic it is," said Darren. "They try to create a bizarre reality out of whatever issue they have attached to. In Tania's case she was going to save the world. People who suffer in this way know they are sinking out of control and start to fight for their lives." There was something dramatically wrong with Tania. She was not taking her anti-anxiety medications anymore. Therefore her manic behaviour couldn't be due to side effects of prescription drugs. He knew he had to get help. He lied and tricked Tania into getting to the Psychiatric Ward of the same hospital where Katherine was fighting for her life.

This time was absolutely terrifying for Darren. He nearly lost his wife. His daughter was in critical condition and in an incubator. Tania was receiving psychiatric care for an illness he did not understand. He knew that things would never be the same and that the problem was extreme. Tania was furious with him for taking her to the Psychiatric Ward and even threatened to divorce him. Somehow he stayed calm and believed that he and his family would overcome this distressing situation. This too would pass. It would require great patience.

The stress in Darren's life was almost unbearable. He had a challenging job and was taking a night class at the time. He was very thankful that his employer was understanding, and gave him the time he needed. Tania was released from the hospital after a two week stay and was joined at home with Katherine three weeks later.

Tania's behaviour and symptoms improved very little during the next ten months. Darren was challenged like never before. Tania was immobilized by Postpartum Depression with Psychosis, the most extreme form of postpartum mood disorders. (For more information see www.pregnancy-info. net/postpartum_psychosis.html). She could hardly take care of herself and Katherine. She was consumed with delusions, manic behaviour and extreme anxiety. Darren had to do virtually everything; as well as working all day he did the night feedings, made meals, cleaned house, did the laundry, etc. Day after day he carried the load. Eventually, Darren became very angry. Why couldn't he rely on Tania for anything? Why couldn't she just get over it?

Tania would constantly call him at work and tell him how she planned to kill him and their daughter. She gave vivid graphic descriptions. She would also talk about killing herself. It was a "living Hell" for Darren. He often left his work and rushed home fearing that an actual tragedy had occurred. The situation became more and more frustrating for him. Darren had grown weary and exhausted himself. It felt like he lived in a fog, just going through the motions of day-to-day living. His physical health deteriorated and his business goals were derailed. He felt like the things he did for his own fun and personal development, were lost. He wondered whether anything mattered anymore. It felt as if the joy within his soul had been robbed. He frequently consoled himself at the end of the day by drinking alcohol.

Why did it have to be this way? It seemed as if his world was deteriorating before his eyes and that there was no way out. He considered taking Katherine and leaving so that he could protect her, but he knew that wasn't the solution. He never even contemplated divorce. It was not an option. Darren comes from generations of married couples staying together. It is the same on Tania's side of the family. No, he would stay "in the battle" and find a way through it. He had to find the courage to continue. He wouldn't run from the problem. Their families helped which was a great relief. "Without the support of our parents who could take over when I couldn't, I truly believe there would have been a funeral in the family. There's no telling what could have happened," Darren reflected.

Tania began to recover from the Postpartum Depression several months later, and started to become her usual vibrant self. She joined a Postpartum Support group and had regular visits her psychiatrist. As they reflected on how this could have happened to Tania, they both looked at the traumatic events leading up to childbirth and the months thereafter. The Postpartum Depression may have been triggered by the trauma of her near death experiences including, alarming high blood pressure and the medications involved with stabilization.

Unfortunately as things got better for Tania, the reverse was true for Darren. He hung in there until the pressure and stress was somewhat released. He was burned out and run down, and now his system was revolting. Darren spiraled down into a depression and was emotionally shutting down. Once again he took time off work, only this time to deal with his own health crisis. It put a tremendous strain on his marriage and family. Tania relied on him for strength and stability. Fortunately Darren knew to seek help and got the help he needed. By talking with close friends and a counsellor, he was able to begin healing and start to enjoy life again.

Darren has been affected by mental health problems in many ways. He has some thoughts on how the medical profession and society can provide better care. He said, "Mental health care is currently being handled with a bandage. It seems that the system is driven to get the patient in, stabilized with medications and then out the door with little to no follow-up. This is what happened in our case. Tania was sent home in a very unpredictable and unstable condition. Like others I have seen, you are left to fend for yourself. The medications greatly helped Tania, but the resulting impact to the family was devastating and heartbreaking. More follow-up care is needed."

'Mental health is greatly misunderstood and under-funded," says Darren. "There is fear that people are just overreacting. If one had a physical illness like a broken arm or infection, there would be no questions asked, but there is resistance today to deal with mental health head on. We need greater acceptance and patience with these problems – we need to realize it affects all of us in some way or another."

What advice does Darren have for others going through this ordeal? He said, "Try not to focus on the negative things going on around you. Our potential to deal with adversity is much greater than we realize. Ask for the help you need. Don't let your ego get in the way. A lonely wolf is very hungry. Be prepared to swallow your pride to help your family. It amazed me to see how when you share your grief and situation with other men in a sincere way, they will drop everything to come and help. You don't have to do it alone," Darren reassures. "And remember you are not the only guy out there experiencing problems, stuff is happening to everyone at some level." Darren went on and said, "Take pleasure in the small things in life like rocking your daughter to sleep, achieving your goals and taking time for yourself. Be willing to be open and honest about yourself – be transparent and real."

"When you almost lose the things that matter most, you realize how little the problems really are – family, love and health are the most important." Darren went on and reflected, "I still have a beautiful family, including a wonderful daughter. This experience has only enhanced my ability to deal with the issues of life and keep what matters most as my highest priority. There may be scars and our marriage was definitively affected with some resentment, but I have to say that we are a stronger family than ever before. We are more grounded, mature and settle disputes much quicker. We appreciate each other."

Conclusion

These stories have demonstrated the importance of openness and understanding in relationships. The people in these stories have shown tremendous courage and tenacity. It is often difficult to perceive what is going on in the minds of others. Some of the most obvious challenges for the husbands surrounded the comprehension and acceptance of what could possibly paralyze their wives so deeply in this postpartum state. These were not the women they had married. All three husbands said how frustrating it was to see their partners dive into a low place where self-pity was prevalent. They would have respected their wives more, if they would have only taken charge of their problem and asked for help earlier. Of course, the husbands now have a greater understanding of how griping Postpartum Depression is, and how impossible it was for the women' to have that level of strength during their darkest days.

It was evident to me by hearing about the support these men gave and the actions they took, that they had a deep desire to hold the family together, somehow, and cope with this destructive illness. Their love for their children was undying. Their inner strength is incredible.

Curtis, Ward and Darren, "bravo" to your bravery and thank you for sharing your truths!

Chapter Five

The Great Debate
To have or not have another baby

The debate about whether or not to have another child should be discussed by the couple and with medical professionals, when Postpartum Depression was experienced with a previous baby. In the book "Conquering Postpartum Depression" [1] it states that the chance of having Postpartum Depression with future children could be as high as 80%. It is an emotional subject and a common source of anguish for many couples.

The three mothers featured in "The Smiling Mask," Carla O'Reilly, Elita Paterson and Tania Bird recently debated the issue which was facilitated by Peggy Collins.

Peggy: So, ladies, now that you have gone through this ordeal, would you have another child? We will start with you, Elita.

Elita: I have been thinking a lot about this (she nervously chuckled). The first thing that comes up is that I feel "gun-shy." I feel like I am still just unravelling from all of this, this mess, and that I'm just making sense of it now. I can still feel that pain and anxiety, and I just think, my first gut reaction is, "no." The only way I think for us to have another child is by accident. Ward has already voiced his opinion, and it's "no" as well, so the decision is made. I could never do this without his support, nor could I ever force it upon him or put him into a position like that. I know that Ward feels that I have a limited threshold for anxiety and stress. My life is a lot simpler with just one child. I have learned that I need to live a simpler life. I am more honest with myself now. What I choose to do with my life has to mean something to me. With that said, I need balance, otherwise it is Ella and Ward that suffer. They feel the stress and frustration too. My goal is for Ella to have a "happy" mom.

Tania: A good wife?

Elita: Yes, and a good wife. I am searching for contentment. Contentment is the key!

Peggy: I believe that acknowledging that threshold and how it affects ourselves and those around us, is part of being a good wife and good mother.

Elita: Talking to my doctors, psychologist and homeopath have all helped me to see the bigger picture of who I am and what I can be. I have been busy cultivating my thoughts and what I can do to become my best. I want to be the best for myself, my husband and my Ella. I also know that I don't want to have another child just to prove to myself that I can do it.

Carla: That is right. Mothers will tend to think that it will be better the next time. I can beat this if I do have a reoccurrence of Postpartum Depression. That is what some people think. I don't want to have another child for that reason.

Peggy: Ok, how do you handle the pressures of having an only child?

Elita: That has been a source of concern, not a big amount of concern though, because Ella has seven cousins and they are all in the city. She is also in daycare at the YMCA with Katherine, (Tania's daughter). They are friends. We have a neighbour boy whom she is friends with, too. So, my concern is not about her being alone. We will even bring a friend with us on holidays sometimes. Ella is not alone. She should not feel alone.

Tania: That is a good strategy.

Elita: We just need to keep Ella's life filled with opportunities to play with other kids. Because she is in daycare she has to learn to share (chuckle). She has already proven that she is capable and she is just over two. It is really not a concern. I am more concerned about me being available to her!

Peggy: Elita, I can see your dedication to doing a good job with the child you have. If you had multiple children it would be harder.

Elita: And I also want to be available to Ward. That is my priority. Our relationship is prime.

Tania: It is interesting that you say this because I am the opposite side of this spectrum. When I close my eyes, I always envisioned four kids. That is not going to happen, but I do believe I will have another one. And, (pause), I also think about the future, specifically when I close my eyes. When Darren and I do this, we see more than one child. So, yeah, I know it is a big leap of faith. I just think it is worth it and if PPD does happen again, it really is only two years of my life to get through. In my case it is a family affair, especially immediate family. If I land in the hospital again, will my family watch Katherine? We've had that conversation already.

Nervous laughter by all .....

Tania: Providing I don't die. I have come close to dying before. The big picture for me is I can have another baby, but I can't handle the stress of a job from 8:00 pm to 5:00 pm. When pregnancy does happen, when I bring another child into the world, I don't want to be at work. I will be a full-time stay at home mom, with a career – doing other stuff that I enjoy.

Peggy: Do you feel that you have healed from the intense level of Postpartum Depression that you had experienced?

Tania: I have done all that I can do. I have talked to many specialists. I joke about getting clearance from them and they all say that I can get pregnant, including specialists, doctors, naturopaths, homeopaths. I think that everything happens for a reason. I had it bad enough the first time that with the second time it won't happen. I have faith. I just want to have another baby. I have no other way to describe it. I feel I need to do it. I need to conquer it.

Peggy: What about you Carla? Would you do it again?

Carla: I have decided that I am not doing this again. My son is four years old. This has been four years of struggle for me. I am finally getting back to being myself again and that feels great. I love my son. I believe that I was given a beautiful boy for a reason; he fulfils me. I don't need another child. This was not an easy decision. When he was two years old, and I started to think about another (child) because everyone else does it at two, yes (pause) I do love babies (pause) but I don't ever want to walk that path again (pause) I can't risk it.

Peggy: To not relive this is the key, isn't it?

Carla: Yes, you need to "get your ducks in a row" before you make a decision. One baby is a hand-full, two children is exponential work. If you are going to do it again, you need to have childcare in place for the other child, right off the start. You would need to have support systems in place, because of the 80% chance of it happening again.

Peggy: So when you think about women who are struggling with Postpartum Depression, what would you tell them? There is always pressure to have another baby.

Tania: Don't rush it.

Elita: You have time.

Carla: Yes, don't rush it.

Elita: Whoever said you need to have kids two or three years apart? Learn about yourself first.

Tania: Yes, know thyself.

Elita: Ward was being told, "You can't only have one child; that is unfair." Yes, you can because you love them. We love her! And there is no guarantee that the siblings will be there for one another.

Carla: It is you as an individual that needs to decide.

Tania: More and more people nowadays are only having one child. People realize how much work it is. They want to put all their energy into one child.

Carla: And do a good job of it.

Elita: And be grateful for it.

Tania: The goal of parenting should be to raise an independent human being. This means different things to everyone.

Elita: And knowing your thresholds, knowing your priorities and living up to them.

Peggy: It is the largest and grandest job we will have in our life.

(Everyone nods in agreement).

Carla: The only way to get healthier is to stop listening to people's negativity. Decide for yourself. You have to live with this decision for the rest of your life. Don't listen to them. If it is negative, it is not true.

Peggy: Don't you feel the pressure?

Elita: It is an old perception. We are so beyond that right now. We are not succumbing. So Tania you feel that you need to have another child?

Tania: Yes, I feel the fear but want to do it anyway.

Carla: You need to have a safety net set up.

Tania: For me, I think, I have come to the realization that life is short, it is but a blink.

Peggy: Because of your near-death experience?

Tania: Yes. Right. I just feel, I want to do this again.

Peggy: Following your heart and intuition?

Tania: Someone logical would say are you insane lady? It just feels like the right thing to do.

Elita: I feel like I am a good enough mother to have more children, but because I am not taking that on, at times I feel like a failure. No, but I am not a failure! I am just listening to my heart and following what feels right.

Carla: The whole perception of being a mother with just one child is often thought as being selfish. You sometimes hear or made, "You are not as good as me because I have three kids!" The mother that has three kids may be tired and worn out. They might not be enjoying themselves. They could be thinking, "I

154

have three kids, I am the mother of the year," but do they really enjoy it? There is a perception that the more children you have the more of a "Super-Mom" you are.

Elita: Yes, there is no right or wrong.

Peggy: I would like to ask this question again for mothers who are currently suffering with Postpartum Depression. What would you say to them when it comes to the pressure of having another child?

Tania: Wait, Wait until you feel better. You have to have children for the right reasons.

Carla: You are in no position to make a decision. Use birth control as soon as possible.

Elita: I agree.

Peggy: I hear you saying that the she should give herself space and time to heal. I can just imagine how getting pregnant again so quickly could magnify the illness, if you did not give yourself time to heal.

(Everyone nods in agreement)

Tania: You could be in a Psychiatric Ward if you pushed it. Time heals all wounds. Wait, don't rush. Every person is different in their healing.

Elita: Also, you would feel angry and resentful. Why would anyone want to bring a child into that kind of atmosphere?

Peggy: To summarize, the key point is that it is an individual decision. Mothers should look deep within themselves and ensure that they are healed. They need to take care of themselves first. We all need to take of ourselves before we can take care of anybody else.

Elita: Some questions you might want to ask yourself, "Are you laughing? Are you happy? Are you sleeping?"

Tania: And consult, consult your spouse, support systems and the medical community. Know full well what you're getting yourself into, with eyes wide open.

Peggy: Yes, eyes wide open. Thank you very much ladies.

This interval was conducted on June 1, 2008. Much growth and healing has happened since.

Chapter Six

Symptoms and Strategies

Most people have heard of Postpartum Depression, but they lack the knowledge and ability to recognize the symptoms. A common reaction of family or friends of someone suffering with Postpartum Depression is to deny or minimize the severity of the symptoms as normal parenting challenges. There are others who suspect that the mother has a serious problem, but they cannot pinpoint exactly what's wrong or how to help. Of course, there are also the mothers themselves who are suffering with this condition. They wonder how to get through it, and what worked for other survivors of Postpartum Depression. How did they climb out of their misery and triumph over it? The objective of this chapter is to offer insight into some of the symptoms of PPD and possible coping skills.

Some Symptoms of Mothers with Postpartum Depression:

1. Insomnia or simply not sleeping well.

2. Severe physical anxiety.
- Feelings of vibration from the inside out.
- Tightness of chest.
- Racing heart.
- Pacing uncontrollably.
- Excessive perspiration.
- Obsessive and/or compulsive behaviours.
- Sensitivity and over-reacting to minor situations with excessive worry.

3. Difficulty calming down.

4. Lack of interest in holding her baby or even naming him or her.
- This may demonstrate a decrease in bonding.

5. Conflicting polarity of emotions, where extreme happiness or sadness is evident.
- Sadness is generally easy to detect. Happiness is less recognizable as a problem because others are delighted that she appears to be bonding with her baby, and is happy. Her happiness is not real and is over-exaggerated.

6. Demonstrates over protectiveness of her baby and paranoia.

7. Displays abnormal personality traits. She is behaving out of character.

8. Displays hysterical behaviour.

9. Demonstrates fits of rage directed at her baby or family.
- This could include yelling, handling her baby in a rough manner, or even not addressing her baby's needs by ignoring her baby (passive aggressive).

10. Hints at suicide and focuses abnormally on death or fears of losing her baby.

11. Loss of interest and motivation and withdrawal from others.

Strategies for Supporting Mothers with Postpartum Depression

These are some of the things we found that were beneficial to us. We hope that friends and families will also use them to help women with Postpartum Depression (PPD).

It is important to convince the mother that it is not a sign of weakness to ask for help! In fact, it is showing responsibility for her well-being as well as her family's. It is imperative that you give importance to her illness and do not minimize, criticize, or ignore it.

Listen, Listen, Listen:

Validate the mother's feelings by asking how she is feeling and show a sincere willingness to just listen. This is very important because some women with PPD are trying to deal with their illness, but are uncertain whether they will be accepted by family and friends. We need to accept PPD as an illness, just like Cancer or Diabetes. Imagine if someone close to you was bed-ridden with Cancer and was also trying to care for a baby. What would you do to help? Listening to sufferers of PPD is paramount. If she contacts you and says that she isn't feeling well or needs a break, do whatever you can to help her. Encourage the mother to seek medical or psychological treatment. When people are desperate they usually show signs of distress (e.g. withdrawn, anger outbursts, feel that others are against them, experiencing fear etc.). It is so important to acknowledge these signs of distress and act!

Seek Treatments:

Encourage the mother or help her to discuss with her doctor, what medications are available and have been successful treatments. Help her research and seek support through alternative methods for self-help, coping skills and other forms of healing processes. When the mother is in the depth of a depression, it is very difficult for her to focus and research solutions on her own. Symptoms of depression include fatigue, low motivation, distrust of others, poor concentration, attention and memory. Remember that once she begins taking medication the side effects may lead to low energy levels. She will need time to rest. Encourage the mother to find a Postpartum Support Group or find one for her! If you have to, attend the first meeting with her!

Grant Breaks:

Give the mother a reprieve from caring for the baby anytime you can. Breaks are very important and they will allow that woman to refresh, recover and reduce worry. Let her choose what she wants to do (e.g. shop, sleep or a pampering activity). Find a trustworthy babysitter so that both parents can have breaks, time to rest and time to reconnect.

People may need to accept that the mom is not able or willing to leave her baby, even for short periods. Be gentle, but do talk about it. It will happen eventually given gentle reassurances.

Ensure the fathers are getting ample support too. Be available to talk with them, in ways that are honest and confidential.

Assist with Chores:

Offer to clean up the house (e.g. wash the dishes, empty the dishwasher, wash clothes, or make a meal). These activities are overwhelming for most new mothers and especially for mothers with Postpartum Depression.

Provide Inspiration:

Encourage the mother with positive energy and inspiration. Send daily inspirational text messages or emails, and buy her light, simple and joyous books or books with inspirational messages, beautiful calendars, relaxation CD's or funny movies. Make her laugh. Give her positive reinforcement everyday and remind her that she is the best mother ever!

Social support for mothers is one of the most important predictors of healing. By supporting mothers with PPD in the ways described, mothers will be encouraged to accept their illness and move towards self-acceptance, self-healing and self-forgiveness!

Strategies for Mothers with Postpartum Depression

These are some of the strategies we did for ourselves and found them to be effective. It is our hope that they will work for others who are suffering with Postpartum Depression.

Understand that you need to use more than one tool or skill to heal yourself for positive long-lasting effects. The more tools you use, the "stronger" you will be! Practicing these techniques with your husband or another support person would make these tools even more "powerful!" These tools help you to let go of guilt! Let it go from sitting on your shoulders, wrenching your gut, squeezing your chest so tight, and the hurting thoughts in your mind. Release the negativity by acting on some of the following strategies that worked for us, and continue to do so.

Take responsibility for Your Health:

Seek medical or physiological treatment first. If you find your doctor or counsellor is not helping, let him or her know. Be "persistent" and find one that resonates with you. Discuss medications with your doctor and which have been successful for others. You can also research alternative or complementary therapies like naturopathy, homeopathy, acupuncture, therapeutic touch and massage, Quantum Biofeedback, Angel Therapy counselling, Bodytalk, and Emotional Freedom Techniques (EFT) etc.

Talk, Talk, Talk:

Talk to whoever seems supportive, and will listen with a compassionate heart. You know you've found someone when the person can simply sit and nod her or his head in acknowledgement, and say you're still the best Mom for your baby.

163

Marriage and Personal Counselling

Professional counselling can be very helpful in facilitating recovery. Counsellors are objective and trained to help patients reflect on past traumas, low self esteem and marital issues. Counselling can be especially helpful for husbands. They may not be comfortable sharing problems with family and friends. Consider marriage counselling together and separate counselling for each other.

Nurture Your Self-esteem:

We have discovered that a low-self image determines how quickly you heal. There are many available programs that teach you how to nurture a healthy self-image. Ask your counsellor or psychologist or support group leader which programs work best.

Relinquish Control:

Other people can most certainly take care of your baby, as well. In fact, it's good for your baby to experience other people.

Gratitude:

Write down what you are thankful and grateful for every day, even if they seem insignificant things. Maintain an attitude of gratitude. By doing this simple action, you will only attract more goodness to you!

Honour Your Individuality:

Do not compare yourself to other mothers! Do not compare your baby or child to others! Honour yourself and your baby by accepting who both of you are and your unique gifts. Use discretion when reading books on parenting. Some encourage the "perfect mother" in unrealistic ways. Respect your instincts as well, and follow through with them to learn what works for you and your baby.

Deep Belly Breathing:
(Adapted from Conscious Breathing; Hendricks, 1995.)

Healthy breathing is a powerful tool. It has a direct effect on our stress levels. When we breathe diaphragmatically we immediately begin the process of increasing our oxygen intake and reducing our body's tension.

When we are in danger our body responds with restricted breathing through shorter and shallower breaths situated more in the upper chest. Our body's automatic response to a threat is to prepare to fight or run. Adrenaline courses throughout bloodstreams, digestion slows and energy is diverted to our muscles. If we continue to breathe shallowly after the danger has passed, through habit or in response to ongoing stress, we deprive ourselves of a return to a fully relaxed state. We alter our body's response to stress through our breathing.

Breathing practice – How to do it!

Pay attention to your breathing. Place one hand on your upper abdomen, the other on your chest. Take a full, deep breath in and notice whether your abdomen rises. If it doesn't and your upper chest and shoulders rise noticeably, expel the breath and this time, when breathing in, push out your stomach to release your diaphragm allowing your lung to fill completely. As you breathe in, your chest and shoulders should stay almost still. As you exhale, your belly settles inward. You may need to practice this way of natural, relaxed breathing a few times. Watch yourself breathe in front of a mirror. Remember, you want to see your shoulders and upper chest remain almost still, while you feel your upper abdomen moving outwards as you inhale and then relaxing inwards as you exhale.

Practicing conscious <u>diaphragmatic breathing</u> can:

- Reduce your immediate and habitual stress levels
- Loosen and relax your sore muscles, especially those in your upper back, chest, shoulders and neck reducing stress related headaches
- Enhance mental concentration and increase physical health
- Face and manage your emotions without repressing them
- Contribute to ongoing health and well-being through simple self-care

Take 2-3 tummy breaths, 12-15 times per day: when you wake up, before and after you eat, when waiting in a line, at red lights, when you look at the time, during TV commercials, when you're feeling frustrated or angry or bored or unhappy. To relax your autonomic nervous system: lengthen your exhalations and shorten your inhalations: inhale (count 1, 2, 3) and exhale (count 1, 2, 3, 4, 5). Find your own best rhythm. To energize lengthen inhalations and shorten exhalations.

Compiled by Maureen Murray, MA. 2004

Postpartum Depression Support Groups:

Consider joining a Postpartum Depression Support Group where support and educational information on PPD is given. These settings not only validate what you're going through, but everyone works toward moving forward. There is much power in a group setting!

Meditation and Prayer:

Meditate and pray anytime you get the chance. Even if you only have 30 seconds or one minute's worth to spare, they add up in a day! Repeat a phrase or word like, "breathe in, breathe out" or "I am surrounded by God's love" or "Ohm!"

Sleep:

Sleep is crucial for a healthy mind and body, without it we are unable to function. Continued unrest can cause depression. Sleep deprivation is a form of torture! As mothers, we need to remind ourselves that rest is important and naps are natural. Healthy amounts of sleep help us perform as caregivers for our children.

Exercise:

Move your body! Get those endorphins moving around in your brain! Get a mini-trampoline for your family room. Stretch your body out. Walk, do yoga, or bicycle. Exercise has been known to reduce low to moderate levels of depression.

Forgive Yourself:

Allow yourself to understand that you're going through a substantial change for a purpose, and learn how to stop operating out of fear-based emotions (e.g. guilt, hate, anger, jealousy, self-doubt, anxiety, uncertainty, etc). You have to learn how to operate out of love-based emotions (e.g. compassion, self- acceptance, contentment, joy etc.) by:

- Feeling the emotion in the moment, and then forgiving yourself by even simply saying, "I forgive myself of the (negative emotion) I'm feeling right now."
- Envision this feeling leaving your body – just let it go!
- Repeat as many times as needed until you feel relief.

This process encourages healing by making room for positive feelings to rise up. It's to raise your awareness. Operating out of love allows you to feel relief and that is vital for good health.

Books and Movies:

Read positive book and watch positive movies like "The Secret" by Rhonda Byrne, "You Can Heal Your Life" by Louise Hay, "The Power of Positive Thinking" by Norman Vincent Peale, and "The Moses Code" by James F. Twyman. Even having one of these movies playing in the background would make a difference. You'll catch certain phrases that may give you that "aha" feeling and it helps when the music is uplifting.

Journaling:

Journal your own story, write about your positive intentions. Pour your feelings out so that you can move forward with the healing process and forgive yourself.

Set Yourself up to Win:

Surround yourself with "balcony" people – people who are your cheerleaders, people that encourage you! Reduce or lose your connection with "basement" people – people who just don't know how to be supportive or positive. Sometimes these people are in your family. It's acceptable to limit your time with these people. It's for you and your child's well-being. "Basement" people could certainly benefit some of these listed techniques!

Thoughts are Powerful:

Realize just how powerful your thoughts are. Your life as of today is a result of your thoughts from the past – imagine what kind of future you can create! Think positive thoughts and good intentions! Visualization and affirmations are effective tools. Visualize a "stop sign" when you're angry, having invasive thoughts or repeating negative self-talk. Immediately replace these thoughts with positive affirmations so that you are changing the "old programs" in your head!

Speak Up:

Use your voice for what it was intended...to speak! Admit you need help and accept support! Be clear and focused on the type of help you need. Make a list. Is it someone coming to clean your bathroom, or doing your laundry or taking your baby for an hour or two so that you can refocus or just relax? Is it someone to just listen? If you want your husband to be more helpful, then describe in detail what that help looks like to you.

You are Number One:

Remember, you are number "one" in your baby's eyes! Hold your index finger up, point it to yourself, and repeat "I am number one" until you believe it.

Reduce Worry:

To curb worrying, ask yourself, "What is the probability of this negative situation really happening?" In all likelihood, the probability will be less than one percent.

Eat Healthy:

Eat as healthy as you can. Introduce more fresh and raw foods into your diet and drink six to eight glasses of water per day to help flush the toxins out of your system.

Supplements:

Take Vitamin B supplements with your doctor's recommendation - vitamins B1, B2, B3 and biotin serve to produce energy, vitamin B6 is essential for proper metabolism, and Vitamin B12 and folic acid play a lesser role in cell division.[1]

Role Model:

Find a role model or confidant when you are emotionally stronger who can mentor you on your healing journey.

Music:

Dance and sing to music with your child! Music has healing properties.

Read:

Read aloud a lot to your child. The rhymes will soothe the both of you as would singing lullabies. Plus, you're doing something together.

Dates:

Plan outings every day, especially in the morning so that you are forced to get out of bed (e.g. coffee with a girlfriend or relative, breakfast, a walk, anything to get your day started). Creating a routine will bring stability to your situation.

Feel Attractive:

Do things for yourself that make you feel attractive. Do your hair and makeup, long soaks in the tub and wear something other than spandex!

Remember, it is natural to have relapses on your healing journey. You just have to "stand right back up" and be positive with yourself, again. Keep moving forward by practicing the tools until they become second nature! And they will!

Notes and References

Preface References:

1. American Psychiatric Association (1994). Diagnostic and statistical manual of mental disorders (4th Ed.). Washington, DC: Author.

2. Pearlstein, T. (2008). Perinatal depression: Treatment options and dilemmas. Journal of Psychiatry and Neuroscience, 33, 302-318.

3. Da Costa, D., Dritsa, M., Rippen, N., Lowensteyn, I., & Khalife, S. (2006). Health-related quality of life in postpartum depressed women. Archives of Women's Mental Health, 9, 95-102.

4. O'Hara, M. W., Zekoski, E. M., Phillips, L. H., & Wright, E. J. (1990). Controlled prospective study of postpartum mood disorders: Comparison of childbearing and nonchildbearing women. Journal of Abnormal Psychology, 99, 3-15.

5. Weinberg, M. K., Tronick, E. Z., Beeghly, M., Olson, K. L., Kernan, H., & Riley, J. M. (2001). Subsyndromal depressive symptoms and major depression in postpartum women. American Journal of Orthopsychiatry, 71, 87-97.

6. Grace, S. L., Evindar, A., & Stewart, D. E. (2003). The effect of postpartum depression on child cognitive development and behaviour: A review and critical analysis of the literature. Archives of Women's Mental Health, 6, 263-264.

7. Murray, L., & Cooper, P. J. (1997). Postpartum depression and child development. Psychological Medicine, 27, 253-260.

8. Lyons-Ruth, K., Wolfe, R., & Lyubchik, A. (2000). Depression and the parenting of young children: A making the case for early preventive mental health services. Harvard Review of Psychiatry, 8, 148-153.

9. Weinberg, M. K., & Tronick, E. Z. (1998). The impact of maternal psychiatric illness on infant development. Journal of Clinical Psychiatry, 59 (Suppl 2), 53-61.

10. Lovejoy, M. C., Graczyk, P. A., O'Hare, E., & Neuman, G., (2000). Maternal depression and parenting behavior: A meta-analytic review. Clinical Psychology Review, 20, 561-592.

11. Martins, C., & Gaffan, E. A. (2000). Effects of early maternal depression on patterns of infant-mother attachment: A meta-analytic investigation. Journal of Child Psychology and Psychiatry, 41, 737-746.

12. Weinberg, M. K., & Tronick, E. Z. (1998). Emotional characteristics of infants associated with maternal depression and anxiety. Pediatrics, 102 (Suppl E): 1298-1304.

13. Carter, A. S., Garrity-Rokous, F. E., Chazan-Cohen, R., Little, C., & Briggs-Gowan, M. J. (2001). Maternal depression and comorbidity: Predicting early parenting, attachment security, and toddler social-emotional problems and competencies. Journal of the American Academy of Child & Adolescent Psychiatry, 40, 18-26.

14. Kurstjens S., & Wolke, D. (2001). Effects of maternal depression on cognitive development of children over the first 7 years of life. Journal of Child Psychology & Psychiatry, 42, 623-636.

15. Hays, D. F., Pawlby, S. Sharp, D., Asten, P., Mills, A., & Kumar, R.

16. (2001). Intellectual problems shown by 11-year-old children whose mothers had postnatal depression. Journal of Child Psychology & Psychiatry, 42, 871-889.

17. Romano, E., Tremblay, R. E., Farhat, A., & Cote, S. (2006). Development and prediction of hyperactive symptoms from 2 to 7 years in a population based sample. Pediatrics, 117, 2101-2110.

18. Sohr-Preston, S. L., & Scaramella, L. V. (2006). Implications of timing of maternal depressive symptoms for early cognitive and language development. Clinical Child & Family Psychology Review, 9, 65-83.

19. Miller, L. J. (2002). Postpartum depression. JAMA, Journal of the American Medical Association, 287, 762-766.

20. Beck, C. T. (1996). Postpartum depressed mothers' experiences interacting with their children. Nursing Research, 2, 98-104.

21. Sinclair, D., & Murray, D. (1998). Effects of postnatal depression on children's adjustment to school. British Journal of Psychiatry, 172, 58-62.

22. Smith, M., & Jaffe, J. (2007). Postpartum Depression. Signs, symptoms and help for new moms. http://www.helpguide.org/mental/ postpartum_depression.htm. Accessed on September 23, 2008.

23. Hay, D. F., Pawlby, S., Angold, A., Harold, G. T., & Sharp, D. (2003). Pathways to violence in the children of mothers who were depressed postpartum. Developmental Psychology, 39, 1083-1094.

24. Goodman, S. H., & Gotlib, I. H. (1999). Risk for psychopathology in the children of depressed mothers: A developmental model for understanding mechanisms of transmission. Psychological Review, 106, 458-490.

25. Weissman, M. M., & Jensen, P. (2002). What research suggests for depressed women with children. Journal of Clinical Psychiatry, 63, 641-647.

26. Josefsson, A., & Sydsjo, G. (A follow-up study of postpartum depressed women: Recurrent maternal depressive symptoms and child behavior after four years. Archives of Women's Mental Health, 10, 141-145.

27. Fletcher, R. J., Matthey, S., & Marley, C. G. (2006). Addressing depression and anxiety among new fathers. The Medical Journal of Australia, 185, 461-63.

28. Schumacher, M., Zubaran, C., & White, G. (2008). Bringing birth-related paternal depression to the fore. Women and Birth, 21, 65-70.

29. Ramchandani, P. Stein, A., Evans, J., & O'Conner, T. G. (2005). Paternal depression in the postnatal period and child development: A prospective population study. Lancet, 365, 2201-2205.

30. Downey, G., & Coyne, J. C. (1990). Children of depressed parents: An integrative review. Psychological Bulletin, 108, 50-76.

31. Condon, J. T., Boyce, P., & Corkindale, C. J. (2004). The First-Time Fathers Study: A prospective study of the mental health and wellbeing of men during the transition to parenthood. The Australian and New Zealand Journal of Psychiatry, 38, 56-6.

32. Egeline, R. M. (2007). Identifying risk factors for postpartum depression. PhD Dissertation, Alliant International University, Fresno, California, USA.

33. Epperson, C. N. (1999). Postpartum major depression: Detection and treatment. American Family Physician, 59, 2247-2254

34. Registered Nurses' Association of Ontario. (2005). Interventions for Postpartum Depression. Toronto, Canada.

35. Engle, G. L. (1977). The need for a new medical model: A challenge for biomedicine. Science, 196(8), 129-136.

36. Zaers, S., Waschke, M., & Ehlert, U. (2008). Depressive symptoms and symptoms of post-traumatic stress disorder in women after childbirth. Journal of Psychosomatic Obstetrics & Gynecology, 29, 61.67.

37. Forty, I., Jones, I., Macgregor, S., Ceasar, S., Cooper, C., Hough, A., et al. (2006). Familiality of postpartum depression in unipolar disorder. Results of a family study. American Journal of Psychiatry 163, 159-1553.

38. Trealor, S. A., Martin, S.G., Bucholz, K. K., Madden, P. A., & Heath, A. C. (1999). Genetic influences on post-natal depressive symptoms: Findings from an Australian twin sample. Psychological Medicine, 19, 645-654.

39. O'Hara, M. W., & Swain, A. (1996). Rates and risk of postpartum depression: A meta-analysis. International Review of Psychiatry, 8, 37-54.

40. Beck, C. T. (2001). Predictors of Postpartum Depression: An Update. Nursing Research 50, 275-285.

41. National Institutes of Health. (2005). Understanding postpartum depression: Common but treatable. http://www.newsinhealth.nih.gov/2005/doc/olfeatures_02.htm. Accessed Sept. 24, 2008.

42. Henshaw, C. (2003). Mood disturbance in the early pueperium: A review. Archives of Women's Mental Health, 6(Suppl 2), 533-52.

43. Henshaw, W., Foreman, D., & Cox, J. (2004). Postnatal blues: A risk factor for postnatal depression. Journal of Psychosomatic Obstetrics and Gynecology, 25, 267-272.

44. Segal, Z. V., Williams, J. M. G., & Teasdale, J. D. (2002). Mindfulness-based cognitive therapy for depression. A new approach to preventing relapse. New York: The Guilford Press.

45. Bledsoe, S. E., & Grote, N. K. (2006). Treating Depression during pregnancy and the Postpartum: A preliminary meta-analysis. Research on Social Work Practice, 16, 109-120.

46. Miller, L. J. (2002). Postpartum Depression. JAMA, The Journal of the American Medical Association, 287, 762-765.

47. Reinecke, M. A., & Freeman, A. (2003). Cognitive therapy. In A. S. Gurman & S. B. Messer (Eds.). Essential Psychotherapies. Theory and Practice (2nd ed., pp. 224-271). New York: The Guilford Press.

48. Stuart, S., & Robertson, M. (2003). Interpersonal psychotherapy: A clinician's guide. London: Oxford University Press.

Chapter **1**	Page 24	1. "Conquering Postpartum Depression – a proven plan for recovery": Ronald Rosenberg, M.D., Deborah Greening, Ph.D., James Windell, M.A., 2003
	Page 25	2. "What to Expect When You're Expecting": Heidi Murkoff, Arlene Eisenberg and Sandee Hathaway, B.S.N., 2002
	Page 28	3. "Conquering Postpartum Depression – a proven plan for recovery": Ronald Rosenberg, M.D., Deborah Greening, Ph.D., James Windell, M.A., 2003
	Page 34	4. "Conquering Postpartum Depression – a proven plan for recovery": Ronald Rosenberg, M.D., Deborah Greening, Ph.D., James Windell, M.A., 2003
	Page 54	5. "The Secret": Rhonda Byrne, 2006
	Page 55	6. "Never Give Up – Ted Jaleta's Inspiring Story": Deanna Driver, 2006
Chapter **2**	Page 63	1. Wikipedia, the Free Encyclopedia; en.wikipedia.org/wiki/Doula
	Page 63	2. Wikipedia, the Free Encyclopedia; en.wikipedia.org/wiki/Meconium
	Page 67	3. http://www.answers.com/topic/thrush-4
	Page 71	4. Dr. Harvey Karp, "The Happiest Baby on the Block," 2003, New York, NYC pages 94-98
	Page 83	5. www.babycentre.com
	Page 84	6. www.dictionary.com
	Page 85	7. "Solve Your Child's Sleep Problems": Dr. Richard Ferber, 2006
	Page 90	8. "The Secret": Rhonda Byrne, 2006

Chapter

3

Page 107   1. "What to Expect When You're Expecting":
Heidi Murkoff, Arlene Eisenberg and Sandee
Hathaway, B.S.N., 2002

Page 125   2. "The Secret": Rhonda Byrne, 2006 and
"You Can Heal Your Life": Louise Hay, 1999

Chapter

5

Page 149   1. "Conquering Postpartum Depression – a
proven plan for recovery": Ronald Rosenberg,
M.D., Deborah Greening, Ph.D., James
Windell, M.A., 2003

Chapter

6

Page 169   1. The Fit Fuel Blog
http://www.fitfuel.com/blog/2008/03/28/vitamin-b-benefits/

Acknowledgements

Carla O'Reilly

"The Smiling Mask" began as a dream of mine three years ago when I was journaling about my experiences and I began to write my story. It was the most healing and effective therapy I could have ever tapped into! I believe that my journey was a gift to create awareness and allow many people to learn from my struggles and survival. I hope this record of my life will inspire other women who may be suffering from Postpartum Depression, to ask for help, talk about their pain, and begin their healing process.

We have to maintain hope because we are the givers of life; we have created the children of the future. These children will be looking to us for wisdom and guidance. They need to know that even though their mothers struggled with Postpartum Depression, they are all wonderful mothers trying to do their best every day.

This story is dedicated to my son, Cameron, who has been in my heart since the moment he breathed life inside of me. I believe God was watching over me and gave me an Angel baby, who was a delight and the "apple of my eye." Every night I kiss him and feel thankful that I have such a beautiful boy. He always seems to amaze me with his brightness and character. Despite my secret illness, I know that I did something right, and that was the way that I loved him.

I would like to thank my husband, Curtis, who after five rough years was able to remain my friend, and be the first to accept my illness, not knowing the long journey ahead of us. He remained strong throughout unbearable periods of my battle and cared for my son, and myself. I know our love for our son is immense; and together we have created a beautiful, healthy, and spirited being.

I would like to thank my Angels and friends, Tania, Elita, and Peggy, who have helped me to believe in my story and in my dreams. You have shown me the power of positive thinking and what strong, determined women can accomplish! Your strength and character will forever remain in my heart.

I would also like to thank my family and friends who have been with me throughout this journey and held my hand through each and every step. You supported me in my darkest hours. I wouldn't be where I am today without you. This also applies to Cameron's amazing grandparents who were always there to help, and to my sisters who always in me believed in me and told me that I was a good mother. Many dear friends carried me when I was far from home and provided guidance, acceptance, a warm cup of coffee and some laughter. I am forever grateful to you for helping me realize the truth in the statement, "it takes a village to raise a child." You allowed me to destroy my mask and accept my illness and heal. I will never forget your friendly faces and warm hearts!

I hope that this book will raise universal awareness that the human spirit is fragile and without the touch of human kindness, we are alone and all wear THE MASK! Reaching out for assistance is not an expression of weakness. Empathy and compassion are the very heart of our existence, and together we will create a universe to fulfill God's vision.

Elita Paterson

I wouldn't be writing these acknowledgements if it wasn't for Tania's encouragement to write my story. I wouldn't be writing my "truth" if it wasn't for Carla's whole-hearted acceptance of me on the team. I wouldn't be writing my story if it wasn't for Peggy's belief in our passion to inspire healing, hope and harmony for families. Thank you so much to each of you for believing in me, which further instilled belief in myself.

I was also able to write my "truth" because of the past and current supports in my life! To my grandparents, thank you for your honesty, strength of character and passion for what you believe. These traits are what I admire most about you, and what I admire most in myself and others. To both Ward's and my parents, your unconditional love and generosity is what truly kept and keep Ward, Ella and I standing tall and strong. To my brother, I love you and think of you everyday. My wishes for you and your family are health, wealth and happiness ~ may you find your peace, too.

I want to send out an immeasurable "thank you" to my extraordinary friends whose unshakable support throughout the years has encouraged me to be the person I am today. I would like to graciously thank my spiritual-mentor, Tim Rezansoff, for teaching me to think differently about ways of the world. To my Director and co-workers, you all have been a source of comfort and validation since I began working with you exceptionally talented and considerate people! To Danita, who shared her thoughts about my story, edit after edit, with such empathy and intensity.

To Sally Elliott, an Angel on earth, who supports families with such vigour and care, and truly listens with her heart. With admiration, I thank Nancy Jane Wells who founded the intensive personal growth program that changed my life; our Marriage Counsellor – Dr. James Pappas; my Homeopath – Dr. Hoe Mark; my Angel Therapy Practitioner – Bonnie Bogner, and my Registered

Massage Therapist and dear friend – Karry Sali ... you all brought me to a place in my life where I am able to transform myself even more to create a life of joy and peace.

Then, there's my husband, my "Wardnick." You are my rock and my safe place to "be." Your ability to remain honest with me is vital to our healthy and ever-growing relationship. Your decision to stand beside me and share our stories could not be more of a testament of how much we have healed, together. We have flourished into two people who can stand their ground and be content with our choices and the consequences. And, because of our experiences I fully believe that Ella will have the tools to live her life with much joy! My hope is that Ella doesn't have to rely on a mask to get through life.

My dearest Ella Bella ... I had wished for you for quite some time, my "Pum'kin!" I have never felt the kind of love that I feel for you. How tremendously honoured I am to have you in my life. My greatest gift in return will be to continue evolving into my highest good so that I can be the best mom for You!

Carla and Curtis, Tania and Darren, Peggy and Jay, Ward and all our Little Miracles ... I cannot express well enough in words what it has meant to me to share such profound growth in such a brief amount of time. Writing and publishing this book has given me the opportunity to be honest about my life journey and growth. It is my hope that others are inspired by my message and find more and more ways to live their highest potential.

Thank you, Thank YOU, THANK YOU!
Elita (aka Linka)

Tania Bird

First and foremost I would like to thank God, the All Knowing, for giving me the grace and courage to write this book about Postpartum Depression. It has been a "topsy-turvy" ride full of emotions and many tears were shed in the writing of my truth. It is but through God's loving acceptance that I share these words with you in the hopes that you too will benefit and find comfort in the knowledge that you are not alone. Postpartum Depression can be overcome. I sincerely hope that my story will provide you with hope, healing, and inspiration.

I would like to thank Sally Elliott for the wonderful support system she provides for new mothers at the YMCA. Your frankness, openness and sharing spirit have helped many women throughout the years, I being but one.

To my husband and life partner, Darren: Thank you and God bless you. Our tumultuous journey was shared together. This has deepened the love and commitment between us. You never gave up hope. It is our belief, that if a couple can survive Postpartum Depression, they can survive anything. From our wedding vows, "Darren, you are the one person I can always turn to, whether it is to share heartache or joy. You rejoice in my successes and applaud my efforts. You know just what to say to me even in my darkest moments and there were many along the journey. You believe in me and encourage me. You accept my faults and my quirks unconditionally. You are perfect for me and when I am with you, I am the grandest vision I have ever held of myself."

To my wonderful and amazing daughter, Katherine, thank you for surviving and thriving despite my illness. I love you more with each passing day. I hope that someday, you will read this book, reflect on your childhood and say it was not so bad considering all things.

To the strong and amazing support systems that I enjoyed and experienced during the last two years – my family, friends, other courageous women, doctors, nurses, psychologists, and psychiatrists: THANK YOU with all my heart.

Peggy Collins

It has been a great honour to be a part of "The Smiling Mask" team as their publisher and mentor. I send my heartfelt thanks to my co-authors and now friends, Carla O'Reilly, Elita Paterson and Tania Bird. You have brought sparkle and joy into my life. Your tremendous commitment to bettering the world by helping others has only increased my commitment to do the same. I have so enjoyed and admired your positive attitude and belief in the divine purpose of this project.

As well I want to thank the husbands for trusting me and openly sharing their stories, so that the male perspective could be represented. Your words will reach, the sometimes forgotten heroes in all of this, the men who generally hold up the fort and the family, while trying the best they can to fix the problem and bring peace to their world. Other men going through similar situations will only be helped and consoled by the chapter we created together. Congratulations to all three of you for achieving a great feat by conquering Postpartum Depression, and growing positively into the people you are today.

I would also like to thank several people who contributed to the editing of this book. We asked readers to provide feedback through an editing process. Their attention to detail and broad perspective were gratefully appreciated and very helpful. Thank you to Rhonda Barry and Paul Barkman. I would like to give special mention of our contributing editor and author of the Preface, Marlene Harper PhD (Psych), MA (C. Psych). Her assistance enriched "The Smiling Mask" with professional strength and clinical information that validates and supports the women's stories and the book's mission.

Tania was the first to approach me about possibly becoming the publisher of this book for their group. I have to be honest, when I first heard of the subject, like the majority of people in our society, I thought about how uncomfortable it is to face the problems of mental illness, and how depressing a subject like Postpartum Depression might be. Did I really want to go there?

Yet something stirred within me to look further and understand what was driving these women to follow their instincts so diligently. The energy around the group was phenomenal. I prayed about it and received my answer. There was no way that I couldn't do it. The stories have to be told; families have to be saved from the silent agony, and at times, the deadly results. Trust me on this one, God is not happy with how we handle Postpartum Depression today. We need to increase awareness and provide more support.

Finding inner peace at any level is progress. There is a positive in every negative situation. The obvious learning and growth these women and their husbands have experienced is definitely a positive life event for all to admire.

Come unto me, all ye that labour and are heavy laden, and I will give you rest
– Matthew 11:28

"Who looks outside, dreams. Who looks inside, awakens," by Carl Jung.

The Smiling Mask
Truths about Postpartum Depression and Parenthood

To Order More Books

Contact

To the Core Consulting
P.O. Box 37016
Regina, SK
S4S 7K3
Canada

Email: info@thesmilingmask.com

www.thesmilingmask.com